SUPPORTING CHILDREN AND THEIR FAMILIES FACING HEALTH INEQUITIES IN CANADA

Edited by Miriam J. Stewart

Supporting Children and Their Families Facing Health Inequities in Canada fills an urgent national need to analyze disparities among vulnerable populations, where socio-economic and cultural factors compromise health and create barriers.

Offering solutions and strategies to the prevalent health inequities faced by children, youth, and families in Canada, this book investigates timely issues of social, economic, and cultural significance. Chapters cover a diverse range of socio-economic and cultural factors that contribute to health inequality among the country's most vulnerable youth populations, including mental health challenges, low income, and refugee status. This book shares scientific evidence from thousands of interviews, questionnaires, surveys, and client consultations, while also providing professional insights that offer key information for at-risk families experiencing health inequities. Timely and transformative, this book will serve as an informed and compassionate guide to promote the health and resiliency of vulnerable children, youth, and families across Canada.

MIRIAM J. STEWART is a professor emeritus in Faculty of Nursing at the University of Alberta.

Supporting Children and Their Families Facing Health Inequities in Canada

Edited by
MIRIAM J. STEWART

UNIVERSITY OF TORONTO PRESS
Toronto Buffalo London

ISBN 978-1-4875-0605-6 (cloth)   ISBN 978-1-4875-3320-5 (EPUB)
ISBN 978-1-4875-2407-4 (paper)   ISBN 978-1-4875-3319-9 (PDF)

Library and Archives Canada Cataloguing in Publication

Title: Supporting children and their families facing health inequities in
   Canada / edited by Miriam J. Stewart.
Names: Stewart, Miriam (Miriam Joyce), editor.
Description: Includes bibliographical references and index.
Identifiers: Canadiana (print) 20210164360 | Canadiana (ebook)
   2021016462X | ISBN 9781487506056 (cloth) | ISBN 9781487524074
   (paper) | ISBN 9781487533199 (PDF) | ISBN 9781487533205 (EPUB)
Subjects: LCSH: Public health – Social aspects – Canada. | LCSH: Equality –
   Health aspects – Canada. | LCSH: Social status – Health aspects – Canada. |
   LCSH: Ethnicity – Health aspects – Canada. | LCSH: Health status
   indicators – Canada. | LCSH: Health services accessibility – Canada.
Classification: LCC RA418.3.C3 S87 2021 | DDC 362.10973 – dc23

University of Toronto Press acknowledges the financial assistance to its
publishing program of the Canada Council for the Arts and the Ontario
Arts Council, an agency of the Government of Ontario.

Canada Council   Conseil des Arts
for the Arts   du Canada

ONTARIO ARTS COUNCIL
CONSEIL DES ARTS DE L'ONTARIO
an Ontario government agency
un organisme du gouvernement de l'Ontario

Funded by the   Financé par le
Government   gouvernement
of Canada   du Canada

Canada

This book is dedicated to my amazing daughters: Evelyn Stewart, MD, FRCPS, who contributed the significant chapter on supporting children vulnerable to mental health challenges; and Shauna Stewart Anderson, MCS, LLB, who offers innovative support programs for refugee and low-income mothers and children.

To my awesome grandchildren: Aidan Stewart Anderson, Chiara DeMarni, Noah Stewart Anderson, Emanuelle Stewart Ouellette, Lorenzo DeMarni, Gabrielle Stewart Ouellette, Samantha Rose Larabie Anderson, Luca McKamey-DeMarni, Hunter James Larabie Anderson, and Thea Stewart Anderson in Heaven (she had just turned 10 and already supported vulnerable people of all ages, including her grandmother!).

To my inspiring parents: Ross and Dorothy Mortimer who were exceptional role models in supporting vulnerable children, adolescents, and parents; and recipients of Caring Canadian Awards.

"The poverty of being unwanted, unloved, and uncared for is the greatest poverty."
— Mother Theresa

"Love your neighbour as yourself."
— Mark 12:31

"As long as poverty, injustice and gross inequality persist in our world, none of us can truly rest."
— Nelson Mandela

"Seek justice, encourage the oppressed."
— Isaiah 1:17

Contents

List of Figures and Tables   xi

Acknowledgments   xiii

1 Introduction – From Isolation to Inclusion:
Diminishing Inequities   3
MIRIAM J. STEWART

Section I: Children's Experiences

Section I Introduction: Children's Experiences   15
JOCELYN EDEY

2 Indigenous Children Coping with Environmental
Health Risks   17
MIRIAM J. STEWART AND SHARON ANDERSON

3 Health Inequities Facing Children Vulnerable to Mental
Health Challenges   29
CLARA WESTWELL-ROPER AND S. EVELYN STEWART

4 Mental Health Risks among Immigrant and
Refugee Children in Canada   66
BUKOLA SALAMI, DOMINIC A. ALAAZI, AND CARLA HILARIO

Section II: Adolescents' Experiences

Section II Introduction: Adolescents' Experiences   81
JOCELYN EDEY

5 Low-Income Adolescents Living with Respiratory Challenges   83
MIRIAM J. STEWART

6 Fostering Support for Indigenous Adolescents Facing Health
Inequities   92
MALCOLM KING AND ALEXANDRA KING

7 Supporting Refugee Adolescents   101
MIRIAM J. STEWART AND JOCELYN EDEY

Section III: Parents' Experiences

Section III Introduction: Parents' Experiences   121
JOCELYN EDEY

8 Low-Income Parents and Caregivers of Children Affected by Health
Challenges   123
MIRIAM J. STEWART

9 Indigenous Parents and Caregivers Caring for Children with
Chronic Health Conditions   135
MIRIAM J. STEWART AND R. LISA BOURQUE BEARSKIN

10 Innovative Programs for Parents Coping with Health Inequities:
Informed by Research Insights   150
NICOLE LETOURNEAU AND MIRIAM J. STEWART

11 Conclusion – Insights and Implications for Future Directions   159
MIRIAM J. STEWART

References   169
Contributors   227
Index   233

Figures and Tables

Figures

3.1 Social determinants of health affecting course and
    management of OCD   45
6.1 Ethical Space   94
6.2 Two-eyed Seeing: *Etuaptmumk*   95
6.3 Trauma-based, resilience-informed model of
    Indigenous health   97

Tables

3.1 Determinants of Health Affected by OCD Symptoms   44
3.2 Aspects of OCD Affected by Specific Social Determinants
    of Health   47

Acknowledgments

This book would not have been possible without the superb contributions of Dr. Dominic Alaazi, Dr. Lisa Bourque Bearskin, Jocelyn Edey, Dr. Carla Hilario, Dr. Alexandra King, Dr. Malcolm King, Dr. Nicole Letourneau, Dr. Bukola Salami, Dr. Evelyn Stewart, and Dr. Clara Westwell-Roper.

The research reported in many chapters was supported through my Senior Scholar and Senior Investigator Awards from the Alberta Heritage Foundation for Medical Research, as well as individual study grants from the Canadian Institutes of Health Research, Social Sciences and Humanities Research Council of Canada, AllerGen NCE, and numerous national and provincial research funders.

Special thanks to Jocelyn Edey for her skill in coordinating communications for this book. We gratefully acknowledge the exemplary contributions of Dr. Michael Kariwo, Dr. Edward Makwarimba, Dr. Sharon Anderson, Dr. Knox Makumbe, Dr. Jeff Masuda, Alison Barnfather, Bronwyn Shoush, Roxanne Blood, Amber Ward, Erika Ladouceur, Phillip Deng, Marwa Alshara, Amanda Almond; numerous research assistants; peer and professional mentors; interdisciplinary research teams; investigators, including Dr. Linda Reutter, Dr. Anne Neufeld, Dr. Edward Shizha, among others; and partner organizations to the success of studies shared in this book. We greatly appreciate the thousands of Indigenous, immigrant, refugee, and low-income children, adolescents, and parents who participated in these nationally funded studies and generously shared their life experiences and insights.

It is gratifying to acknowledge the University of Toronto Press's support for publishing this text.

Finally, I am grateful for the superb supporters in my life and for the love of God and Jesus Christ.

SUPPORTING CHILDREN AND THEIR FAMILIES
FACING HEALTH INEQUITIES IN CANADA

1 Introduction – From Isolation to Inclusion: Diminishing Inequities

MIRIAM J. STEWART

Gaps and Goal

Research reveals social isolation and significant gaps in social support for vulnerable children, youth, and their families facing health inequities. There is currently little capacity in health-relevant systems in Canada to address these health inequities through targeted supports. Indeed, "income-related health inequalities have persisted despite Canada's publicly financed universal health care systems" (Canadian Institute for Health Information [CIHI], 2016, p. 17), contributing to disparities that remain a national concern. These disparities are not randomly distributed. Specific subpopulations suffer a burden of illness and distress greater than other residents of Canada. Indigenous[1] peoples, newcomers,[2] the poor, the homeless, children and youth in disadvantaged circumstances, and people with poor literacy skills are populations that are more likely than others to become ill and less likely to receive appropriate health services. The wealthy live longer than the poor, and experience fewer chronic illnesses, and lower levels of mental distress (Beiser &

---

1 "Indigenous" is a non-legislated term used throughout this book to acknowledge the First Nations, Inuit, and Métis as distinct Peoples with historical and ongoing connections with the Canadian territory, and recognize self-determination to define themselves. The term "Aboriginal" will be used when referencing legislation and previous articles and reports.
2 "Newcomer" is a term used through chapters in this book that refers to immigrants (persons coming to live permanently in a foreign country), migrants (persons moving to another country in order to find work or better living conditions), and refugees (persons forced to leave their country in order to escape war, persecution, or natural disaster). Each term will be used when referring to a specific group (e.g., teen refugee in chapter 7).

Stewart, 2005). Despite commitments to equity and access to health and health care, 16.8 per cent of Canadians live in poverty (Citizens for Public Justice [CPJ], 2018). Health, education, and legal systems have not kept pace with demographic shifts and growing geographic inequality in child and adolescent health needs. Moreover, child health inequities are created, sustained and aggravated through multiple, related pathways (Pearce et al., 2019). Social and structural determinants, including insufficient quality education, few employment opportunities, and inequitable gender norms have diminished adolescents' prospects for health (Azzopardi et al., 2019).

Processes that lead to the unequal distribution of social determinants of health reinforce the need for "a more detailed understanding of *why* children from less advantaged backgrounds have worse health and, from an intervention perspective, *how* policies and *interventions work*, for *whom* and under *what circumstances*" (Pearce et al., 2019, p. 5, emphasis in original). Although research has documented health disparities within and across countries, there is an urgent need nationally to analyze disparities among vulnerable populations in children, adolescents, and parents; describe mechanisms through which factors such as poverty compromise health; illuminate barriers; and test programs that reduce their inequities and isolation.

Given these research gaps, the goals of this book are to (1)share research insights from studies designed to promote inclusion and social support, enhance health equity, and reduce isolation; (2) identify timely issues of social, economic, and cultural significance; (3) communicate scientific evidence, professional knowledge, and experiential knowledge of affected children, youth, and parents/family caregivers; (4) offer keen insights into life for children, youth, and families experiencing health inequities; (5) inform intervention strategies to support vulnerable children, adolescents, and families; and (6) identify implications for programs and policies.

Studies conducted in Canada, by Canadian multidisciplinary research teams, peer reviewed by Canadian experts, and funded by leading refereed research organizations are described. Collectively, they comprise hundreds of hours of interviews, questionnaires, and surveys with thousands of participants across Canada, representing a diverse range of socio-economic and cultural backgrounds, thereby offering comprehensive yet nuanced insights into life of children, adolescents, and their parents who are vulnerable to health inequities.

This book synthesizes insights from the authors' previous research, alongside other published work to illuminate broader problems pertinent to health equity in Canada. It moves beyond simply describing problems and prevalence to offering solutions and strategies. This book will serve as an informed and compassionate guide for students and professionals to help vulnerable children, youth, and families facing inequities in Canada.

Theoretical Foundations

This book is guided by key theories focused on social support, social networks, social isolation, social exclusion, coping, and resilience. Pertinent social science concepts inform many book chapters. Social support is a resource for coping with challenges and includes interactions with family members, friends, peers, and professionals that communicate information, affirmation, practical aid, or understanding (M. Stewart, 2000).

Social determinants of health, such as social support, have informed the studies shared in this book. These are the conditions in which people are born, grow, live, and work, shaped by the distribution of money, power, and resources (including income, education, employment, and ethnicity), and are linked to physical and psychological health inequities (Government of Canada, 2018a; World Health Organization [WHO], 2019). Specific social determinants of *child health* encompass socio-economic, cultural, political, and physical climate; living conditions; community; household resources; parents and caregivers; parenting and child health behaviours (Pearce et al., 2019). Variables that influence social support encompass socio-economic status, culture, age, gender, and ethnicity (Gottlieb & Bergen, 2010; Jones, 1998).

Income as Health Equity Determinant

A recent editorial in the *Lancet* journal, "Tackling the Multidimensionality of Child Poverty" (2019), underscores that "poverty and its associated risk factors in childhood have extensive consequences," which have the potential to affect health and productivity through adulthood (p. 199). Significant health inequalities have been observed for those with low socio-economic status. Health outcomes worsen progressively with lower socio-economic status (Government of Canada, 2019). Income is one of the most important health determinants because purchasing power affects a wide range of risk factors. Increasing income equality (i.e., decreasing gap between the rich and the poor) by raising the income of those most disadvantaged can improve health, aid in the reduction of health inequalities, and enhance population health (Lynch et al., 2004). Higher income determines living conditions, such as safe housing

(Government of Canada, 2013), and increases control. Indeed, there is compelling evidence that higher social and economic status is associated with better health (Government of Canada, 2013). The Canadian Medical Association (CMA) observes that socio-economic factors are more significant for creating or damaging health than either biological factors or the health care system (CMA, 2017).

Poverty involves social, political, and cultural marginalization, which exerts negative impacts on self-worth, spiritual vitality, and well-being. Many factors beyond income separate the most vulnerable from the least, including discrimination, disability, ethnicity, and socio-economic norms (Williams et al., 2016). Individuals who face multiple barriers have increased vulnerability to poverty. A recent report identified key demographics of people in Canada who have particularly high poverty rates using the Census Family Low Income Measure: 19.6 per cent of children, 36 per cent of single parent families, 23.6 per cent of Indigenous peoples, and 20.8 per cent of racialized people (CPJ, 2018). The prevalence of working poverty is significantly higher among Canadians who have not completed high school, First Nations people living off reserve, recent immigrants, and racial minorities (Government of Canada, 2018b).

Our previous research (M. Stewart, Makwarimba, et al., 2009) revealed that poverty inhibited participation in social organizations and social gatherings that foster feelings of acceptance and a sense of community. We found that low-income people experienced greater isolation and less sense of belonging than higher-income people (M. Stewart, Reutter et al., 2007). Poverty also shapes lower-income people's perceptions and experiences of being stigmatized, avoided, and isolated (M. Stewart, Makwarimba et al., 2009). Material deprivation can generate social exclusion and isolation because of limited resources for engaging in community, leisure and family activities and for accessing health and social services (M. Stewart, Anderson et al., 2008).

Chapters 5 and 8 in this book examine the cycle of poverty and health problems facing many adolescents and parents living with a low income in Canada. The dual stigma associated with poverty and chronic illness in adolescents is explored, as well as associated isolation from peers and desire for social inclusion. Low-income parents' and family caregivers' sense of helplessness, frustration, and fear were investigated. Interventions designed for low-income adolescents and parents, focused on reducing isolation and filling support gaps in their coping repertoire, are also presented in these chapters. In chapter 3, influences of social determinants such as income and ethnicity for vulnerable children's mental health are examined.

Ethnicity and Cultural Determinants

Culture and ethnic origin influence inequities in health, and access to and quality of health and social services. Negative effects are especially evident for racialized and Indigenous peoples, as well as those at the lower end of the social gradient (Canadian Public Health Association, 2018). Some people face health risks determined by dominant cultural values that contribute to the perpetuation of marginalization, stigmatization, loss or devaluation of language and culture, and lack of access to culturally appropriate health care and services (Government of Canada, 2013). To illustrate, parents of children with functional disabilities, from ethnic or racial minorities, with low incomes, or limited English-language skills are most likely to report deficient relationships with health service providers (Deatrick, 2017).

Intractable conflicts and violence have led to expansion in the number of refugees around the world, with women and children comprising an extensive segment (International Organization for Migration, 2018). Since 1990, the number of international migrants escalated from 153 million to 258 million in 2017. In the same time period, the number of migrants living in Canada increased from 4,333,318 to 7,861,226, representing a 49 per cent increase (United Nations [UN], 2018). The health challenges of these migrants and refugees are critical and highlight the importance of "allowing migrants unfettered access to health care" ("Refugee Health Is a Crisis," 2019, p. 2563).

Immigrants and refugees are marginalized when their efforts to overcome key settlement challenges are impeded (Government of Canada, 2015). Moreover, new immigrants to Canada are more likely to face barriers to accessing health care services (Government of Canada, 2015). Our previous research revealed many uncertainties and challenges facing newcomers in Canada, including language barriers, unemployment, underemployment and attendant poverty, perceived discrimination and racism, support deficiencies, isolation, and inadequate access to services (M. Stewart, Anderson et al., 2008). "Reform and renewal initiatives regarding immigration, employment, social services, education, justice and health have not been sufficiently attentive to the culturally-embedded support needs of immigrants and refugees" (M. Stewart, Anderson et al., 2008, p. 152).

In this book, chapter 2 highlights environmental health inequities experienced by Indigenous children. The importance of culturally appropriate services, and Indigenous health indicators are emphasized in chapter 6, which explores upstream determinants of health such as connectivity to culture, language, and land. Chapter 4 shares insights from studies of immigrant and refugee children, specifically children from Africa. Significant discrimination and differences in service uptake among ethnic groups resulting from a complex interaction of language barriers, cultural beliefs, illness stigma, financial resources, and social resources are presented in this chapter. The cultural and social impacts of an accessible technology-based support intervention for Syrian refugee adolescents are reported in chapter 7. Chapter 10 emphasizes culturally influenced support deficits of parents living in vulnerable circumstances (e.g., refugee new parents).

Social Support as a Health Determinant

The World Health Organization's Commission on Social Determinants of Health (CSDH, 2008) and the Chief Public Health Officer's *Report on the State of Public Health in Canada* (Public Health Agency of Canada [PHAC], 2008) reinforced the relevant role of social support as a key social determinant of health, a health promotion mechanism, and a protective factor in resilience. Resilience can be experienced through a reciprocal process that utilizes different sources of support (Ungar, 2018). Interactions and relationships with social network members can be supportive or non-supportive, and can exert positive or detrimental effects on physical, psychological, and spiritual health (M. Stewart, 2009).

Social exclusion and social isolation have been associated with poor health outcomes and are entangled with other social determinants of health, such as ethnicity and income (Andermann, 2016; Marmot, 2007; Raphael, 2007). Inadequate incomes can prevent people from participating in social activities and restrict their ability to access and retain social support, leading to social isolation (Hawthorne, 2006). Income challenges and changing help patterns in Indigenous communities negatively affect support reciprocity (Richmond, 2007). Stigma linked to income and ethnicity can also foster feelings of isolation (M. Stewart, Makwarimba et al., 2009). Reduction of social exclusion and isolation requires attentiveness to structural barriers; cross-sectoral and non-traditional partnerships (Crombie et al., 2005; Employment & Social Development Canada [ESDC], 2018; Galabuzi, 2005); participation by disadvantaged people in the design and delivery of services (Davies, 2005; McClure, 2000); use of new technology; sustainable and flexible services/programs (ESDC, 2018); and social support strategies (M. Stewart, Makwarimba et al., 2009).

Salient support interventions designed to increase social support and diminish social isolation, and enhance resilience for vulnerable children, adolescents, and parents experiencing health inequities are shared in chapters 2, 5, 6, 7, 9, and 10. Key foundations of these social support interventions were based on social comparison, social exchange, and social learning theories. According to social comparison theory, individuals compare themselves and affiliate with others (e.g., peers in groups with shared language and culture) who have first-hand experiential knowledge of a stressful situation (Borkman, 1999). Social exchange theory asserts that support may involve benefits and costs for both recipients and providers, and if individuals perceive reciprocity in their social relationships, it is more likely that they will value and retain these relationships (Chibucos & Leite, 2005). Social learning transpires when individuals observe others, especially peers, and combines reinforcement with awareness and expectations (Tennyson & Volk, 2015). Peer support, based on personal "experiential knowledge," is a critical source of social learning for vulnerable people and can supplement professional support derived from professional knowledge (Borkman, 1999).

Relevant Research Methodologies and Collaborations

Public participation strategies underpin the success of studies seeking to promote health, health equity, and resilience of vulnerable children, teens, and families. This book shares scientific evidence, professional knowledge, and experiential knowledge of affected children, youth, and families. Indigenous ways of knowing (experiential), participatory action research, community-based participatory research, and strength-based interventions are key methodological approaches addressed throughout the book.

Chapter 6 focuses on resilience of Indigenous youth and introduces Indigenous approaches to research and interventions. Indigenous or traditional ways of knowing is "a way of observing, discussing and making sense of new information" (Berkes, 2009, p. 153). Indigenous knowledges are living ways of making sense of the world rooted in community practices, rituals, and relationships (Ontario Institute for Studies in Education, 2020). A related approach is *Etuaptmumk* – Two-eyed Seeing, referring to learning to see from one eye with the strengths of Indigenous knowledges and from the other eye with the strengths of Western knowledges, and learning to use both these eyes and ways of knowledge together (Institute for Integrative Science & Health, 2018). Such views are supportive of Indigenous research and interventions that contribute to connectivity with culture, language, and land; restoration of positive Indigeneity; and self-determination.

Mixed-methods and participatory action research (PAR) designs were utilized for many studies presented in this book. Consistent with principles of community engagement in participatory action research (Vaughn et al., 2013; Bergold & Thomas, 2012; Lesser & Koniak-Griffin, 2013), capacity building and collective understanding were emphasized. Community-based participatory research is particularly pertinent for addressing influences of social determinants of health (Cargo & Mercer, 2008) and offers community members opportunities to become involved in each step of the research process (Ellis et al., 2007).

The reduction of health inequities demands interdisciplinary, multi-sectoral, and multi-site perspectives due to complex relationships among social determinants of health (M. Stewart, Makwarimba et al., 2007). Our research teams combined academic and professional knowledge and expertise with experiential knowledge of community members and organizations. Authors of this book represent diverse disciplines and areas of expertise, including nursing, psychiatry, public health, human ecology, and medicine. In research reported in this book, participation of multiple stakeholders ensured relevance of studies to the complex needs of people living in poverty, Indigenous peoples, and newcomers; and to those who enable accessible services and supports for vulnerable people. Moreover, incorporating low-income, immigrant, refugee, and Indigenous people as interviewers enhanced data validity; built individual and community research capacity; and fostered empowerment. Impressive benefits of involving vulnerable community members experiencing health inequities included increased appreciation for research, insights into vulnerable populations' service preferences, and cohesiveness of support provision. Input from service providers, grounded in their experience of working with vulnerable groups, enhances researchers' capacity to develop contextually and culturally appropriate strategies.

Our investigators used pluralistic approaches that reflected interdisciplinary inclusiveness, valued participatory approaches to enhance relevance for vulnerable people, and built on both quantitative and qualitative methods. Support interventions aimed at reducing health disparities utilized quantitative and qualitative methods, which supplemented and complemented each other.

It is important to identify factors that mediate effects of diverse risks and stressors, in addition to those that enable health agency (Edge et al., 2014). A strength-based approach (exemplified in peer-support interventions in this book) can be effectual in creating and maintaining hope and well-being in people (Jafari, 2017). Health in populations strengthens resilience and social cohesion, empowers people, and contributes to social capital (WHO, 2018).

Our research programs also emphasize translation and transfer of evidence to public, practice, and policy domains. For example, knowledge translation strategies for vulnerable parents of children coping with health inequities are described in chapter 10.

Structure and Sequence

This book communicates relevant recent research on accessible sustainable programs designed to support children, youth, and parents coping with health disparities. Special attention is given within each life stage to individuals from vulnerable groups with chapters focusing on low income, immigrant and refugee, and Indigenous children, adolescents, and their parents/caregivers. This life stage approach enables the presentation of challenges, risks, and factors that influence individuals at various periods of life. For example, a child's experience living with issues associated with asthma (e.g., not participating in sports) is quite different from their parents' experiences (e.g., difficulties paying for medication). The approach presents a picture of challenges and opportunities for growth across various stages of life. Examining the experiences of different age groups within a similar context can inform the development of interventions and services that address specific and relevant health, social, and economic circumstances of individuals and groups (see section introductions for more information).

Consistent with this life stage sequence of content, three chapters following the introduction focus on children, the next three chapters on adolescents, and the final three chapters, prior to the conclusion, on parents and family caregivers. Congruent with the theoretical foundations, different social determinants of physical and/or psychological health are highlighted. All book chapters emphasize social support and pertinent conceptual premises, including social isolation. Within the initial section, chapter 2 focuses on a physical health condition (asthma) and influences of ethnicity and other relevant salient determinants for Indigenous children. Chapter 3 offers a comprehensive analysis of ethnicity and other social determinants on mental health of children and teens. Chapter 4 pays particular attention to ethnicity influences on the mental health of refugee children from Africa. The next section, centred on adolescents, is introduced by chapter 5, which examines the experiences of adolescents living in poverty with challenges of a chronic physical health condition. Chapter 6 emphasizes culturally appropriate care and health equity for Indigenous adolescents, with an examination of promising support interventions. The final chapter of this section presents a support intervention designed for Syrian refugee adolescents and explores impacts, insights, and implications. Chapter 9 transitions to another life-stage section focused on parents and family caregivers of vulnerable children and adolescents. This chapter presents the unique challenges facing Indigenous parents and family caregivers of children with chronic health conditions. Chapter 10 provides a review of programs developed to address the support needs of four different vulnerable groups of parents, including refugees from Sudan and Zimbabwe, and highlights the importance of knowledge translation. The book concludes with chapter 11, which underscores the implications of studies shared in the preceding chapters for services, programs, and policies supporting vulnerable children, adolescents, and families.

Important impacts of social determinants of health and health disparities affecting vulnerable children, adolescents, and parents in Canada are highlighted throughout this book. Common health inequities, explored in this book, illuminate challenges and intervention opportunities to support these children, youth, and parents. Social isolation, loneliness, lack of belonging, exclusion, and gaps in support are often experienced, and magnified in vulnerable Indigenous, newcomer, and low-income populations. Social support, like socio-economic status and ethnicity, is a significant social determinant of health. Moreover, socio-economic status, gender, ethnicity, and age influence social support resources. Support interventions shared in this book primarily focus on reducing social isolation and loneliness; improving support seeking as a coping strategy; increasing inclusion; alleviating stress; and enhancing health behaviours and health services use.

Interdisciplinary collaboration and public participation strategies underpin the success of reported studies seeking to understand challenges, and promote health, strength, and resilience for vulnerable children, teens, and families. This book relays recent research testing innovative interventions to support children and families vulnerable to health inequities in Canada.

SECTION I

Children's Experiences

Section I Introduction:
Children's Experiences

JOCELYN EDEY

Economic inequalities that include housing problems, school challenges, and treatment access increase risks for children. Immigrant children's risks revolve around culture, racism, and social class. Indigenous children also encounter cultural and socio-economic risk factors. This section will highlight social determinants, such as ethnicity, that influence both children's mental and physical health challenges and the experiences of children vulnerable to health inequities.

The first chapter in this section, "Indigenous Children Coping with Environmental Health Risks," will present stressors and struggles facing Canadian Indigenous children affected by respiratory health conditions, as an example of prevalent physical health challenges. Focusing on early childhood development and care is critical as Indigenous peoples are the youngest, fastest growing population in Canada facing environmental health problems, and Indigenous children are especially vulnerable. Studies will be highlighted to share the complex cultural challenges facing Indigenous children and parents living with respiratory health challenges. Following an examination of environmental risk factors and support needs, culturally relevant interventions designed in response to insights and experiences communicated by Indigenous children and their parents will be shared.

The second chapter of the children's section, "Health Inequities Facing Children Vulnerable to Mental Health Challenges," will introduce social factors influencing childhood mental health. The chapter explores social, familial, and biological determinants influencing children's mental health in general, and in a common childhood-onset psychiatric disease: obsessive compulsive disorder. Experiences of living with childhood mental health problems and the roles of families are discussed. Comprehensive analyses of impacts of social determinants, including socio-economic status and ethnicity on child mental health, and conversely impacts of mental health conditions on social determinants such as education, occupational functioning, and marital status are shared. The authors' studies examined numerous intervention strategies to help children and their families cope. Inequities in interventions and barriers to services are also illuminated. Finally, implications for practice, programs, and policies and ideas for further research are highlighted.

Chapter 4, "Mental Health Risks among Immigrant and Refugee Children in Canada," concludes this section and will explore mental health problems experienced by a specific vulnerable population in Canada: immigrant and refugee children. This issue is timely as Canada currently has the highest percentage of immigrants among the G8 countries, children are overrepresented in refugee and immigrant populations across Canada, and the risk of mental health problems for immigrant/refugee children and youth is higher than for older immigrants. Research evidence suggests that refugee and immigrant children suffer elevated levels of emotional problems; a health disadvantage attributed to pre-migration experiences of conflicts and post-migration experiences of racism, discrimination, and poverty. This chapter outlines the current state of evidence on the mental health of immigrant and refugee children in Canada and identifies implications for mental health policy and practice.

This section addresses the multiple, intersecting social determinants that affect the mental and physical health experiences of children. Reducing inequities during early childhood requires a multilevel, multifaceted response (Moore et al., 2015). By examining factors such as ethnicity and its effects on physical and mental health, we can enhance the health of children and their futures.

2 Indigenous Children Coping with Environmental Health Risks

MIRIAM J. STEWART AND SHARON ANDERSON

A World Health Organization report contended that investment in children can reduce health inequities in Indigenous populations (Nettleton et al., 2007). Nevertheless, disparities in Indigenous children's health outcomes persist (Halseth & Greenwood, 2019) despite advances in medical technology and increased global wealth (Victorino & Gauthier, 2009). Focusing on childhood is critical as Indigenous peoples are the youngest, fastest growing population in Canada, and Indigenous children are an especially vulnerable portion of this population. Distinct structural, systemic, and environmental factors obstruct Indigenous children's development, including insufficient community-focused, culturally safe and accessible, health, education, child welfare, and social services systems; and policies that influence (un)healthy family or community environments (Halseth & Greenwood, 2019). The aim of this chapter is to share insights and experiences of Indigenous children and their parents affected by increasingly prevalent health problems (Global Initiative for Asthma [GINA], 2020), which will demonstrate the links among ethnicity, socio-economic status, and health inequalities.

Both biological and sociological environmental factors, which include nutrition, allergens (inhaled and ingested), pollutants (environmental tobacco smoke), and microbes, influence the development of asthma (GINA, 2020). In Canada, environmental health risks pose major challenges (Statistics Canada, 2013a), particularly for Indigenous children, inflicting harmful impacts on physical health, psychosocial well-being, and quality of life (Assembly of First Nations, 2007; Chang et al., 2012). Asthma and allergies are among the most common chronic conditions affecting Indigenous children (King et al., 2004; Kovesi, 2012) and adults in Canada (Carrière et al., 2017; Rosychuk et al., 2010a, 2010b), and may be underdiagnosed among Indigenous people in isolated or remote areas (Gessner & Neeno, 2005; Pahwa et al., 2015).

Respiratory system diseases are the leading cause of hospitalization for both Indigenous and non-Indigenous children, but Indigenous children have a hospitalization rate twice has high as non-Indigenous children (Guèvremont et al., 2017). Hospitalization rates linked to asthma and bronchitis among Indigenous children have increased 200 per cent since the 1980s, compared with a 50 per cent increase for non-Indigenous children (Assembly of First Nations, 2007; Boffa et al., 2011). The clinical and economic burdens related to these conditions are significant, and will become more prominent as the prevalence of asthma in Canada continues to increase (Ismaila et al., 2013).

Less than two-thirds of Indigenous children with asthma in Canada – and approximately one-third with allergies – receive the treatment they need (First Nations Information Governance Centre [FNIGC], 2011). This leaves many Indigenous children languishing in a vicious cycle of flare-ups and superficial, short-term solutions. Indigenous children are far more likely to end up at clinics or emergency rooms than specialists' offices (Sin et al., 2002), where root causes can be detected and substantive treatment undertaken. As one child in our research explained: "We had to wait, like, five hours to drive there to a hospital. There was just nothing. There was no clinic either. I didn't have puffers then" (First Nations child with asthma and allergies). The result is inadequate control of the condition, harsher symptoms, and a sicker child. Another First Nations child described the help they received at a physician's office: "There's this one doctor we went to and she just gave us a prescription. She didn't even know what was wrong or anything. She just, like, okay, what do you need today? And then my mom just told her, and she didn't really help ... just got what we wanted."

Given the higher rates of respiratory illness and associated higher health care utilization rates among Indigenous children, risk factors reinforcing inequitable health outcomes require clarification (Crighton et al., 2010; Rosychuk et al., 2010b). Risk factors for Indigenous peoples with asthma encompass genetics (Chang et al., 2012); income; low education (Jetty, 2017; Karunanayake et al., 2019; Kinghorn et al., 2019); environmental factors that include higher exposure to overcrowded housing, poor indoor air quality, and air pollution (Carrière et al., 2017); and inadequate access to culturally sensitive health professionals (Fenton et al., 2012).

What causes Indigenous children to suffer disproportionately with asthma and allergies? Is it a reflection of the higher rates of poverty endemic to Indigenous populations across the country? Low income increases the risk of airway infections that exacerbate asthma and also reduces access to the health system and to diagnosis (Karunanayake et al.,

2019). There are multiple mechanisms by which racism adversely affects health (Williams & Cooper, 2019; Williams et al., 2019). High rates of discrimination based on Indigenous identity are reported (Allan & Smylie, 2015; Browne, 2017; Nelson & Wilson, 2018). The intergenerational connection between ethnic inequities and health outcomes amplifies challenges faced by Indigenous communities (Kopel et al., 2014), including exposure to high-risk environments. Traditional health research glosses over how interpersonal and structural racism experienced by Indigenous people intersects with and increases disproportionate social, economic, and structural disadvantages to increase health inequity (Varcoe et al., 2019).

Our research team spoke with numerous Indigenous children affected by respiratory health problems and their parents, seeking insight into the distinct challenges faced by these vulnerable children and their support needs (M. Stewart, Castleden et al., 2015; M. Stewart, King et al., 2013). These insights can inform the development and delivery of effective, beneficial services, while also removing barriers to service access.

Understanding the Problem

As understanding springs from relationships, our work started by building partnerships with the First Nations and Métis organizations operating in Alberta, Manitoba, and Nova Scotia. Our research team interviewed experts from these groups and created a ten-member Community Advisory Committee. Comprised entirely of First Nations and Métis people, the committee's role was to ensure that our study team asked the right questions; that people's rights and culture were respected; and that the answers sought addressed questions that mattered not just to the researchers but also to the Indigenous communities and people themselves. The Indigenous advisers provided valuable guidance throughout the study, including recruitment.

Once the study's parameters were set and approved by the Community Advisory Committee, it was time to reach out to affected children and their families. To further ensure cultural sensitivity and comprehensive understanding, the research assistants serving as our study's front line – who engaged with participants, conducted individual interviews, and facilitated group interviews – were chosen from affected communities, and represented a broad swath of Indigenous cultures: status and non-status, First Nations and Métis, urban and rural. Our field researchers were thus not simply interviewers, but translators, bridging theories of academia with the discourse of affected community people.

Recruitment began with our Indigenous field workers reaching out to their own communities, across three Canadian provinces (Alberta, Manitoba, and Nova Scotia). They visited schools, community health centres, and childcare providers to distribute flyers and meet with local parents and children, asking if they knew any children with allergies or asthma who might be interested in participating in the study. This technique, called "snowball sampling," enabled the recruitment campaign to extend organically through a larger Indigenous community without requiring vast resources. Researchers speak with a few people, who provide the names of possible participants, who are themselves invited to suggest other people who might join the study. A small cluster of people thus expands into a vast network. To supplement this strategy, field researchers also conducted radio interviews, hung posters in community centres, and advertised in newsletters targeting Indigenous readers. By the time recruitment was completed, forty-six Indigenous children – ages six to nineteen – agreed to partake in the study. The children were evenly divided between boys and girls and identified themselves as Métis, First Nations, or Inuit. All suffered from asthma and allergies, though the extent of their symptoms varied.

All children participated in individual interviews, which were conducted by trained members of our team. Interviews followed a semi-structured guide and interviewers were given leeway to ask follow-up questions, probe carefully for further information, or redirect the conversation if a chosen strategy did not seem to work. Interviews lasted from thirty to sixty minutes and elicited information on Indigenous children's lives, environmental health challenges, and services used to help manage their respiratory conditions. Once the individual interviews were completed, child participants were invited back for second interviews that took place in a group setting. Group interviews lasted for one hour. Building on the individual interviews that focused on life with asthma and allergies, and on services used by these Indigenous children, the group interviews emphasized the services desired and the supports needed by children. The goal of the interviews was to discern experiences, needs, and risk factors for Indigenous children facing environmental health risks.

After all interviews were conducted, audio recordings were transcribed into written reports, and reviewed by the research team to identify recurring themes. Qualitative methods were employed to corroborate, elaborate, illuminate (Bergold & Thomas, 2012; Schulze, 2003), and enhance understanding of meanings and perceptions of support needs, support intervention preferences, and appropriate intervention(s) (Ahmed et al., 2004; Government of Canada, 2014). The team found a complex web of cultural and economic factors. No one strand blocked access to appropriate care, but woven together into a dense mesh, they formed barriers, which many Indigenous children and their families found difficult or impossible to penetrate.

Stigma and Stereotypes

Indigenous children believed they were treated differently from their friends and classmates because of their respiratory health problems. Sports and active play were difficult, and the children struggled to keep up with their peers: "I was bullied at school because I couldn't run. The kids kept chasing me. I couldn't go outside in the spring or fall because of the allergens" (First Nations child). A First Nations child with asthma and allergies explained what happened when he had to treat his symptoms: "When I was a little kid, I felt embarrassed because everybody looked at me when I used ... my inhaler." Moreover, Indigenous children bore the added burden of a culture that clashed with their condition. With their focus on the natural world, many meaningful Indigenous ceremonies cause environmental health risks and play havoc with restrictions linked to allergies and asthma. Rituals often include open fires with heavy smoke, smudging (burning of herbs to bless or cleanse), animal hides, and fur – common allergens in the environment capable of triggering asthmatic episodes in sensitive children. Consequently, Indigenous children can feel cut off from their cultural roots, unable to participate in family celebrations. Even with understanding families, this exclusion can have a profound impact on children's sense of belonging, as activities central to their culture affect them in a visceral, negative way. These cultural ceremonies are less commonly practised in urban settings, but city-dwelling Indigenous children faced their own obstacles. Respiratory conditions often excluded them from school, sports, field trips, and other extracurricular outings. In many cases, Indigenous children believed this exclusion highlighted their minority status, inviting further ostracism.

Isolated

Many children and their parents lacked the social networks and resources which more affluent families take for granted. Although friends offered help; they generally came from the same communities as the children and knew little about asthma, allergies, and treatment strategies. Parents yearned for supportive, informed peers for their children who could guide them, but often such peers could not be found.

In rural communities, poor transportation and long distances in the physical environment made these challenges even worse. Public transit was often non-existent or ran infrequently or at inconvenient hours. Although telephone-based and online health services were available in some circumstances, many children lacked the tools needed to access them as home internet and telephone service were not universal.

Indigenous families living in cities faced their own unique challenges. Services were less remote geographically, however accessing them remained difficult, as many were unaware of resources available or struggled to navigate the system to find them. Health resources were physically closer, but cultural resources seemed more distant, as many Indigenous families felt cut off from the community networks that form a key element of their culture. For example, in many Indigenous communities, Elders are an invaluable and respected source of knowledge and comfort.

Lack of Knowledge

Children's sense of being "lost" was often exacerbated by lack of understanding among their families and peers about asthma and allergies. When asked about these conditions, many struggled to explain exactly what triggered allergies or asthmatic flare-ups, how inflammation affected the lungs in the short and long term, and how these conditions could be managed properly. One First Nations child noted:

> I didn't know a lot. I didn't know who to ask, and there was really nothing out there that I could see that was handy or helpful. All I knew was [that] asthma ... was something with breathing. If you did exercise, you'd have problems breathing, but, I mean, I didn't know it was serious. I didn't know much about it. I just knew you always had it.

Some parents inadvertently adhered to inadvisable practices with their children's medicines, letting kids take them seasonally when they should be taken year-round, or opting for the quick fix of Prednisone received in the emergency room rather than the less powerful – but, over the long term, safer – daily inhaled steroid medicine. A gulf of understanding emerged between parents' descriptions of their children's experiences or the child's understanding and the complex, technical language of health professionals. In many cases, teachers and physicians attributed health-related problems to Indigenous culture, when the immediate issue was the disease itself and the factors that lead to the clinical problems. Indigenous children who missed school or activities were considered lazy; children who were tired or hyperactive were dismissed as undisciplined; and children who struggled with grades or had trouble concentrating due to treatment side effects were marked as unambitious or slow. One mother noted that her son's eczema made socks painful, but his teacher castigated him for going barefoot attributing this to his native culture.

Smoking is more prevalent in Indigenous communities than in the general population, and its constant presence in the environment can pose challenges for children and their families (Jetty, 2017; Pahwa et al., 2017). Keeping households smoke-free can cause stress and friction, particularly when several family members are habitual smokers. Even in households where the family members themselves do not smoke, asking visitors to "butt out" can feel taboo when smoking is considered culturally acceptable. To make matters worse, many children faced significant peer pressure to start smoking themselves.

High Cost of Low Income

Many participants did not have pharmaceutical coverage and children's medications had to be paid out of pocket. Indigenous participants had different levels of medical coverage from employment, provincial plans for people with low income, or the Canadian federal government's Non-Insured Health Benefits program. There are many First Nations, non-status, Inuit, and Métis peoples who have no coverage or who have insufficient health and pharmaceutical coverage. Medications administered in the emergency room, to stabilize children's flare-ups, were available free of charge for children in our studies. In other cases, children rationed their medication, saving inhalers and pills for times when breathing problems were worse.

Lastly, the environment in which many Indigenous children live made them particularly vulnerable to respiratory problems. Many participants described harsh, remote community environments, where allergens and irritants were widespread. Low-income houses on many reserves were underserviced and plagued with dust and mould, further aggravating children's respiratory conditions. Primary contextual factors linked with respiratory health outcomes also include crowding, indoor air quality (e.g., dampness, pets inside home, improper ventilation), and outdoor air quality; Pahwa et al., 2017).

Seeking Solutions

Study interviews yielded a wealth of information regarding beliefs of Indigenous children and their parents about children's lives with asthma or allergies and about the barriers that impeded their quest for happy, healthy lives. The next step was to identify strategies to remove these barriers, or at least shrink them to manageable levels. Consequently, a follow-up study was launched that provided support and education to foster optimal coping skills (M. Stewart, Castleden et al., 2015).

Working in conjunction with Indigenous groups in three provinces across Canada, the study team established a series of programs designed to engage Indigenous children who suffered from respiratory challenges. Although the structure varied based on local needs, the essential plan was the same: create a social support program where children with respiratory problems could interact with one another through a combination of cultural activities, games, and group discussions. The settings ranged from summer camps to community centres. Activities included education, guest speakers, peer mentorship, and peer support interspersed with traditional music and dancing, Indigenous prayer, cooking, arts and crafts, relay races, and sports. The goal was to engage children while imparting vital skills to lead healthy lives and forging supportive relationships with peers. Indigenous peer mentors understood first-hand what it was like to be Indigenous and have asthma and/or allergies.

Responses to the support program were immediate and positive. Younger and older children and adolescents valued meeting peers, whose cultural backgrounds and health challenges mirrored their own, and making friends. More remarkable, they enjoyed the learning activities as much as the games. Many children reported that they understood their asthma or allergies better and learned helpful strategies for coping. Talking about their illness in an open, positive environment helped eliminate shame and fear that had built up in their minds, making them more comfortable sharing with friends and family members.

While the face-to-face peer support-group meetings and camps for Indigenous children were successful, such programs are inherently limited to those who can attend in-person. In our peer support interventions, although programs were offered free of charge, transportation was provided, and organizers delivered the broadest possible outreach; some families still "slip through the cracks." In poor or marginalized communities especially, a child's attendance at a summer camp or peer-support group can be a challenge. To address this issue, a program was piloted that offered an alternative source of support. Unlike programs that required in-person attendance, this program operated entirely online.

The online pilot study began with testing. The study team consulted with health professionals who worked closely with Indigenous communities to gain insight into specific information and services needed by children. They recommended that sessions focus on two key areas: asthma triggers and coping strategies. The former category offered detailed descriptions of common irritants for Indigenous children with asthma or allergies, how they could be identified, and how they could minimize or avoid exposure. The latter category dealt with the skills that Indigenous children with asthma or allergies need on a daily basis. A series of Power-Point slides were crafted regarding identified topics and an Indigenous artist was hired to draw culturally meaningful graphics. Two versions of the slide set were made: one for older children, and one with simpler language for younger children. The research team, which included individuals from Indigenous communities, assessed the team's previously developed workshops and education materials, and revised and adapted them to serve Indigenous children. An advisory committee comprised of Indigenous leaders reviewed the work, ensuring that materials accurately reflected their culture.

For interventions to be effective, engaging informative materials for Indigenous children, and an Indigenous leader capable of bringing the material "to life" are vital. For this reason, the training course for the peer mentors who were responsible for delivering the program received considerable attention. Peer mentors from Indigenous cultures (First Nations, Métis, Inuit) completed two ninety-minute training sessions, in which they learned how to assess group dynamics, encourage brainstorming, facilitate problem solving, help child participants set goals, lead role play, and generate data through field notes and questionnaires after the online support-group sessions.

Support-group meetings were held in a digital real-time environment, allowing children to speak with and see one another using a video interface. Indigenous children were able to talk as a group and were encouraged to discuss strategies for avoiding environmental triggers and overcoming challenges linked to their illness. Under the careful guidance of Indigenous group leaders, these children shared their feelings about life with asthma or allergies, the fears and frustrations that accompanied their conditions, and the people – parents, grandparents, teachers – who helped them. Opening up in front of others helped children accept and understand their illnesses: "I learned that it's OK to talk about your feelings with other people that aren't just your family or your really close friends. You can talk ... with anyone who you know, who you can trust, and who won't make fun of you" (Indigenous child). Indigenous children described times they had been excluded or bullied because of their asthma or allergies, and shared advice on how to avoid or overcome these and other problems, based on personal experience.

Emotional exploration was balanced with practical guidance as children in online groups offered tips on use of inhalers, other treatments, and coping strategies they found useful. Indigenous children felt better informed and supported, and gained a sense of satisfaction from meeting other children who'd faced similar challenges. An Indigenous child explained: "It's pretty fun knowing ... that other people trigger ... to those things like I am [because] I don't know people that have asthma like me. It's nice to hear people say that they have asthma and what their triggers are."

After the online group sessions were complete, nearly all the children who participated provided very positive feedback, and many reported that the support program helped them become more physically active, take their medications more consistently, and improve their abilities to manage challenges.

Insights and Implications

The purpose of these studies was to examine barriers to health services access for Indigenous children with environmental health challenges, and then pilot-test support programs specifically designed to address children and parents' expressed needs. Stigma and racialized stereotyping, inadequate support systems, insufficient knowledge, low income, and harsh environments intersected to increase these Indigenous children's undue suffering with environmental health problems. A single, simple solution would not fit all the needs of Indigenous children with environmental health needs. Rather, a robust network of services and supports was needed to fill gaps commonly faced by Indigenous children in rural First Nations and Métis communities and urban centres.

The concept of intersectionality clarifies how interlocking influencing factors connect to shape experiences (Varcoe et al., 2019). Our studies of Indigenous children's and their parents' experiences demonstrate that focusing solely on single issues may blind providers to the barriers to culturally appropriate health management. Urban Indigenous children and their parents were more likely to identify instances of racism and discrimination when accessing the health system. Children living in rural Métis and First Nations communities felt excluded by traditional Indigenous cultural practices that exacerbated their asthma and allergies. Lack of knowledge about management of their health conditions intersected with poverty, inadequate housing, and harsh rural environments to exacerbate challenges of respiratory health problems. Income deficits and changes in government policy are barriers for Indigenous communities and diminish support exchange (Richmond, 2007).

The Indigenous children participating in our support intervention studies confirmed they became better prepared to manage problems. They credited their increased self-efficacy to Indigenous peer and professional leadership of support groups and to opportunities to communicate with peers. Programs that enhance protective resources such as social support, problem solving, and stress-management skills have been successful in reducing racial health disparities (Cohen et al., 2006; Williams & Mohammed, 2013). Despite reported needs for support from peers in similar situations for Indigenous children/adolescents with respiratory problems (M. Stewart, Castleden et al., 2015), and the importance of peers for Indigenous children (Andersson & Ledogar, 2008), salient support programs engaging peers had not been tested prior to the studies described in this chapter. Moreover, interventions that address the support needs identified by Indigenous children affected by environmental health challenges are exceedingly rare (M. Stewart, King et al., 2013).

Given the multifaceted and systemic nature of racism and health inequities, reducing health disparities of Indigenous children with environmental-related health problems requires ongoing work to improve support and education and address inherent differentials in homes, schools, health systems, and communities. There is now a sizeable body of research that documents the effects of racism on health, and there are intervention studies that point the way for more comprehensive programs (Varcoe et al., 2019; Williams & Cooper, 2019; Williams et al., 2019). More systematic and sustained multilevel (program, policy, cultural) applications of current evidence is needed. It will be critical to consider abundant health and social challenges facing Indigenous children and youth. Endeavours to empower and engage these young people are essential "to normalizing outcomes for the next generations, potentiating decreased health disparities and healthier communities" (Petrucka et al., 2016, p. 191). These outcomes can be facilitated by providing conditions that support early childhood development, including household income above the poverty line, safe housing and communities, ability to afford nutritious foods, and supportive parenting education (PHAC, 2018). Three strategies recommended by Williams and Cooper (2019) represent an optimum path forward:

1) Integrated practice and policy efforts that neutralize the ways racism blocks individuals' access to resources needed to thrive.
2) Initiatives that shift health system's narrow focus on treatment to practices and policies which foreground social determinants of health, prevent disease, and provide high-quality person-centered care tailored to the person's context and culture.
3) New investments to identify optimal strategies that enhance public awareness of the nature and extent of racial inequities and build political will to eradicate racial inequities. (p. 19)

Appreciating variations in challenges and strengths of First Nations, Inuit, and Métis peoples is essential as they reflect their unique histories, languages, cultures, environments, beliefs, and world views in relation to health experiences (Atkinson, 2017). This awareness is critical in development of programs and policies that will support, educate, and care for Indigenous children.

3 Health Inequities Facing Children Vulnerable to Mental Health Challenges

CLARA WESTWELL-ROPER AND
S. EVELYN STEWART

Approximately one in five Canadian children is affected by a mental disorder (Waddell et al., 2019). However, epidemiological survey data suggest that fewer than 40 per cent of these individuals have had contact with mental health care providers, emphasizing significant unmet need (Georgiades et al., 2019). Untreated mental illness in childhood or adolescence may lead to severe and enduring mental and physical health problems in adulthood (Carver et al., 2015). Suicide is the second leading cause of death for Canadian youth, accounting for one in five deaths among young adults between fifteen and twenty-four, with highest prevalence among individuals with mental disorders (Carver et al., 2015). These prevalence estimates point to an urgent need to integrate developmental perspectives in the planning and delivery of mental health services (MacLeod & Brownlie, 2014).

The significant impacts of mental disorders on morbidity, mortality, growth, and development are socially determined, resulting in the highest risk of poor mental health outcomes among members of society experiencing discrimination and marginalization. Both the development and the trajectory of psychiatric diseases are shaped by the social, economic, and physical environments in which children and their families live. This chapter first reviews the most recent data linking social determinants and mental health outcomes among Canadian children and adolescents, and their relevance to vulnerable populations, including children of immigrant and Indigenous families. More work is needed to understand the contribution of individual risk factors to specific mental disorders and how experiences of psychiatric disease are affected by social determinants. To provide an in-depth example (based on the authors' work), the chapter draws attention to obsessive-compulsive disorder (OCD), a common neuropsychiatric condition identified by the World Health Organization (WHO) as one of the leading causes of worldwide medical disability (Murray & Lopez, 1997).

Relatively little attention has focused on the social determinants of illness trajectories in children affected by OCD and their families. Experiences of living with childhood-onset OCD and the roles and experiences of families are discussed through a health equity lens. Accordingly, analyses are provided of the impacts of social determinants including socio-economic position and ethnicity on symptoms and access to care, and, conversely, the impacts of this mental health condition on social determinants such as education, school, family, occupational functioning, marital status, and quality of life. Inequities in interventions and barriers to services are also illuminated.

Social Determinants of Mental Health in Children

Socio-economic Disadvantage

The associations between socio-economic inequalities and mental health problems in children and adolescents have been reviewed previously (Reiss, 2013), including reviews with a specific Canadian focus (Jakovljevic et al., 2016; MacLeod & Brownlie, 2014). Dimensions of socio-economic position as measured in research studies include parental income, education, occupation, and marital status. Factors linked to these dimensions that may mediate the relationship between socio-economic position and mental health outcomes include parental emotional well-being and parenting practices (Bøe et al., 2014; A.E. Russell et al., 2016). Other social risks associated with above-threshold scores on screens for child psychosocial dysfunction relate to caregiver education, employment, childcare, housing, food security, and household heat (Spencer et al., 2020). The Canadian Community Health Survey 2013–2014 provided strong evidence not only for a link between sociodemographic factors and mental health symptoms but also for income-based inequity with respect to mental health care access (Bartram, 2019).

Children living in poverty – as measured by family income, parental employment, and neighbourhood income – are significantly more likely to experience poor mental health compared with peers from families with higher incomes (Jakovljevic et al., 2016). For example, they are three times more likely to meet criteria for a psychiatric diagnosis, including both externalizing disorders (such as ADHD, oppositional defiant disorder, and conduct disorder) and internalizing disorders (such as depression and anxiety) (Boyle & Lipman, 2002; Costello et al., 1996; Waddell et al., 2002). Children from low-income households perform below their middle-class counterparts on tests of intelligence and school achievement (Bradley & Corwyn, 2002), and have also been found to have deficits in working memory, language abilities, and cognitive flexibility compared with their middle-class peers (Farah et al., 2006). Beyond those meeting strict diagnostic criteria for a psychiatric disorder, many additional children experience negative emotional and behavioural responses to family financial insecurity (Jakovljevic et al., 2016). In British Columbia, for example, children with lower household income were more likely to be categorized in lower social-emotional functioning groups when compared to their peers, as measured by the Early Development Index in kindergarten (Thomson et al., 2017).

Recent findings from the Ontario Child Health Study similarly point to an association between poverty and symptoms of externalizing disorders, although children from impoverished households had fewer symptoms when situated in high-poverty neighborhoods (Patten, 2019). More significant problems were identified in children exposed to neighbourhood adversity (Boyle et al., 2019). These findings suggest that children from low-income families are disproportionately harmed by exposure to adversities such as unsafe neighbourhoods. Moreover, environmental factors may differentially affect specific symptoms; for example, a small study of parents attending child and adolescent outpatient services in Kingston, Ontario, found that children with externalizing but not internalizing disorders tended to live with unemployed single parents who had lower education levels and lived in rented or assisted housing (Alavi et al., 2017).

In the UK Millennium Cohort Study, 64 per cent of the total effect of socio-economic conditions on socio-emotional behavioural problems at age fourteen was mediated by early-life factors measured at age three (Straatmann et al., 2019). However, social determinants continue to affect the mental health of adolescents and emerging adults. A Canadian study of youth between fifteen and twenty-four seeking outpatient treatment for substance use, with or without other concurrent mental disorders, found that 80 per cent endorsed a concern with at least one social determinant of health, most frequently being income/finances (Settipani et al., 2018). When youth under the age of thirteen were moved from a high-poverty to a low-poverty neighbourhood, enduring positive effects included lower levels of depression and anxiety (Brent, 2020). Adverse childhood experiences are associated with increased risk of complex physical and mental health disorders later in life (Maunder et al., 2019). The adverse effects of early life stress – including poverty, sexual abuse, physical abuse, emotional abuse, physical illness/injury, death of a family member, domestic violence, and natural disaster – on the risk for mental illness manifest early in development.

Housing

An individual's or family's living environment may independently affect mental health. Data from the 2008 Aboriginal Children's Survey suggests that housing conditions – measured by homeownership and housing satisfaction – are associated with the physical and mental health of young Inuit children, even when sociodemographic factors are taken into account (Kohen et al., 2015). An association between psychosocial and household function also points to the importance of the home environment among low-income children with chronic conditions (Suku et al., 2019).

Street-entrenched youth experience high rates of child abuse history, substance use disorders, and other mental illnesses (Saddichha et al., 2014). Data from the BC Health of the Homeless Study suggest that depression and psychosis are more common than expected among homeless female youth; panic disorder, alcohol use disorder, and cannabis use disorder are common among homeless males (Saddichha et al., 2014). A study of young adults experiencing first episode psychosis in Montreal found that 26 per cent of the 167 participants between eighteen and thirty years of age were homeless at some point (Lévesque & Abdel-Baki, 2019). Those who were homeless were more likely to have a history of child abuse and substance use disorder and had poorer two-year symptomatic and functional outcomes (Lévesque & Abdel-Baki, 2019). At Home/Chez Soi was a large randomized controlled trial of the Housing First model in five Canadian cities, including 164 youth with mental illness between ages eighteen and twenty-four (Kozloff et al., 2016). The study found that these youth had low educational attainment, high rates of substance use disorders and victimization, and high unmet health care needs compared to early adults (Kozloff et al., 2016). Taken together, these Canadian data emphasize the prevalence of homelessness among youth with serious mental illness and the negative impact of being street-entrenched on their disease trajectories.

Geography

Geographic location has been indirectly linked with mental health outcomes. Data from the US National Survey of Children's Health found that parent-reported and doctor-diagnosed mental health conditions were more common in rural compared to urban children; social determinants of health likely accounted for this disparity (Kenney & Chanlongbutra, 2020). Similarly, an Australian study found that children and adolescents from rural areas had poorer mental wellness when compared to a normative sample, and this was attributable to personal and family factors such as low income (Peters et al., 2019). In Canada, internalizing symptoms and suicidality are more common among youth ages twelve to twenty-four in northern regions (Henderson et al., 2017). Mental health diagnoses may also be associated with migration patterns within and between rural communities. For example, a study of children of sawmill workers in Western Canada found that adolescents and young adults who grew up in the same rural community where they were born were at a lower risk of being diagnosed with an acute stress reaction or depression compared to matched controls who had grown up in a different community from their birthplace (Maggi et al., 2010).

A recent Ontario study of community mental health and addictions treatment suggested that community-based services may effectively limit the need for acute hospital-based care, but this was the case primarily in higher-income neighbourhoods and urban areas (Gatov et al., 2020). Rural areas of Ontario, regions with unsatisfactory public transport, and areas with higher levels of socio-economic disadvantage had greater unmet needs for mental health services (Duncan et al., 2020).

Food Insecurity

The Longitudinal Study of Child Development in Quebec (Melchior et al., 2012) showed that children from food-insecure families were disproportionately likely to experience persistent symptoms of depression/anxiety and hyperactivity/inattention (Melchior et al., 2012). After controlling for immigrant status, family structure, maternal age at child's birth, family income, maternal and paternal education, prenatal tobacco exposure, maternal and paternal depression, and negative parenting, only persistent hyperactivity/inattention remained associated with food insecurity (Melchior et al., 2012). This study points to an important and modifiable factor that is likely to affect learning, social interactions, and school success, and is consistent with a recent US study demonstrating an association between food insecurity and attention problems (Spencer et al., 2020).

Selected Populations Differentially Affected by Mental Health Inequities

Children of Immigrant Families

Children in immigrant families have diverse experiences; some families immigrate for economic or educational reasons, while others seek safety from violence or persecution (Linton et al., 2019). The experience of

violence, displacement, and resettlement increases the risk for psychiatric disorders and psychosocial impairment (Hodes & Vostanis, 2019).
Post-traumatic stress disorder and depressive symptoms are found at
higher prevalence in children and youth who have been exposed to
war. Internationally, there is a high level of unmet mental health service
needs for approximately half of refugees who are under the age of eighteen, even in high-income countries (Hodes & Vostanis, 2019).

The 2002 Canadian Community Health Survey suggested that immigrants who arrived prior to age six reported the highest risk for mood
and anxiety disorders compared with those who immigrated at the age of
eighteen or older (Patterson et al., 2013). A Canadian study of children
between four and eleven found that compared with Canadian-born children, those who had recently immigrated were more than twice as likely
to live in poor families, but had lower levels of emotional and behavioural
problems overall (Beiser et al., 2002). Indeed, the mental health effects
of poverty among non-immigrant children were indirect and primarily
mediated by single-parent status, parenting style, parental depression,
and family dysfunction; these factors could not similarly explain the relationship between poverty and emotional problems among foreign-born
children (Beiser et al., 2002). These data emphasize the importance of
specific family contexts in mediating the relationship between poverty
and mental health.

Both pre- and post-migratory factors affect refugee children's emotional regulation during resettlement. The New Canadian Children and
Youth Study, a national study of immigrant children and youth in Canada, identified both migration-specific and universal factors contributing to childhood emotional problems (Beiser et al., 2010). Significant
universal factor predictors included parental depression, family dysfunction, and parental education, while migration-specific variables included
country of origin, region of resettlement, resettlement stress, prejudice,
and limited linguistic fluency (Beiser et al., 2010). Other studies have
identified similar resettlement contingencies contributing to children's
mental health and emotional problems: parental mental health, intra-
familial conflict, settlement stress, and separations from parents (Beiser
et al., 2014). A survey of 103 mothers and their five- to thirteen-year-old
Syrian refugee children resettling in Canada found that children who
more frequently engaged in family routines showed better anger regulation (Elsayed et al., 2019). Greater post-migratory daily hassles were associated with worse sadness regulation for children with lower levels of pre-
migratory life stressors, but not for those who experienced higher levels
of pre-migratory life stressors (Elsayed et al., 2019). A focused ethnographic study in a food bank in Montreal, Quebec, identified challenges

to well-being among families who had been in Canada for between two months and twenty-three years. These included insufficient finances, non-standard work, hurdles in professional equivalency, isolation, children's acculturation, inadequate access to health care, and the Canadian winter (Pitt et al., 2016).

A recent qualitative study identified multiple barriers to mental health care among immigrant and refugee mothers in Edmonton (Tulli et al., 2020). These included financial strain, lack of information, racism/discrimination, language barriers, stigma, feeling isolated, and feeling unheard by service providers (Tulli et al., 2020). On the other hand, facilitators of access to care included services offered for free or by schools and personal levels of higher education (Tulli et al., 2020). Notably, a population-based longitudinal cohort study from 1996 to 2012 using linked health and administrative datasets in Ontario found that rates of recent immigrant mental health service utilization were at least 40 per cent lower than for long-term residents (Saunders, Lebenbaum et al., 2018). The decrease in outpatient mental health visits by immigrants in that study was felt to represent a potential emerging disparity in access to preventative care (Saunders, Lebenbaum et al., 2018). Indeed, immigrant youth were more likely to present with a first mental health crisis to the emergency department than non-immigrants, emphasizing the need to identify mental health problems earlier, prior to crisis, in immigrant populations (Saunders, Gill et al., 2018).

Indigenous Children and Youth

Internationally, Indigenous peoples experience significant inequities stemming from colonial experiences and intergenerational trauma. In Canada, colonization and the legacy of residential schools have also contributed to health disparities among Indigenous children and adolescents, including increased rates of depression, anxiety, conduct disorder, substance use disorders, and suicide. Mental health services are unable to meet current needs (Whitbeck et al., 2008).

A recent systematic review of studies published between 1996 and 2016 included eight Canadian reports that quantitatively evaluated the association between psychosocial variables and mental health among Indigenous children (Young et al., 2017). Children's negative cohesion within their families, the presence of adverse childhood experiences, substance use, experiences of discrimination, co-morbid internalizing symptoms, and negative parental behaviour were associated with negative mental health outcomes (Young et al., 2017). Positive family and peer relationships, high self-esteem, and optimism were associated with increased positive outcomes (Young et al., 2017). Importantly, Aboriginal cultural status among Grade 5 students in Saskatoon, Saskatchewan, was not independently associated with moderate or severe depressed mood after full multivariate adjustment; parental educational status was a confounder, suggesting that mental health disparities may be modifiable by targeting determinants of health such as education (Lemstra et al., 2008).

In a Canadian survey of 1,103 youth accessing homeless services in 2015, Indigenous homeless youth experienced greater rates of mental health and substance use challenges compared with non-Indigenous youth (Kidd et al., 2019). Female as well as sexual and gender-related minority youth (for example, individuals identifying as lesbian, gay, bisexual, asexual, transgender, two-spirit, queer, or intersex) were particularly at risk. Child protection history and street-victimization were especially relevant to current distress levels. These findings emphasize the need for interventions that include prevention initiatives addressing the legacy of colonization (Kidd et al., 2019).

The links among children's familial environments, psychological traits, substance use, experiences of discrimination, and mental health outcomes highlight key targets for more concerted efforts to improve the mental health of Indigenous children (Young et al., 2017). A recent scoping review of mental health services in the Northwest Territories used the First Nations Mental Wellness Continuum and emphasized Indigenous Social Determinants of Health (Elman et al., 2019). Others have focused on school-based interventions for behavioural and emotional challenges (Jack et al., 2020; Maina et al., 2020). Wendt and colleagues (2019) outline the principles of community psychology that can inform community-based research in Indigenous communities: ecological perspectives, empowerment, sociocultural competence, community inclusion and partnership, and reflective practice.

Obsessive Compulsive Disorder: Social and Environmental Risk

The specific ways in which social risk factors affect health are fundamental elements of diagnosis and formulation in psychiatry. Socio-environmental risk factors play a key role in the development, severity, and chronicity of mental disorders, in part because they make engagement with evidence-based interventions more difficult and living with mental illness more challenging (Shields-Zeeman et al., 2019). Many factors beyond medical care quality and access may drive outcomes, including social risk factors associated with neighborhood safety, educational attainment, housing stability, and food security. Whether directly or indirectly, social risk factors shape health, health behaviors, and health services use and costs (Shields-Zeeman et al., 2019).

Conversely, poor mental health can also negatively impact social determinants in a cumulative manner over time (WHO & Calouste Gulbenkian Foundation [CGF], 2014). Living with a psychiatric disorder such as OCD – particularly with childhood-onset OCD – has the potential to impact educational attainment, occupational function, economic security, housing, and relationships. Childhood and adolescence, in particular, are crucial periods during which social determinants contribute to the ways in which psychiatric symptoms develop and are managed. Poorly managed symptoms can cause functional impairment across multiple domains, impede future employment, create barriers to socioeconomic improvement, and increase the risk of physical and psychiatric co-morbidities, including anxiety and substance use disorders (Hale & Viner, 2018; WHO & CGF, 2014).

The remainder of this chapter will review the many impacted aspects of health and development in children with OCD and their families that create unique developmental challenges through adolescence and beyond. While important advances in the neuroscience of OCD have begun to impact clinical formulation and treatment planning (Dougherty et al., 2018), a less appreciated but significant need at the interface of science, medicine, and social policy is to better understand sociodemographic influences on OCD symptoms and barriers to evidence-based clinical care. The following question begs attention: What social factors make a child with OCD more vulnerable to negative outcomes related to both the disease itself and to associated functional impairments?

OCD is a serious mental illness that is both underestimated and poorly understood by the general population and frequently misrepresented by media sources. The diagnosis of OCD requires the presence of obsessions and/or compulsions, *in addition to* significant and negative functional/ emotional impacts. Obsessions are recurrent and persistent thoughts, urges, or images that are experienced as intrusive and unwanted and cause distress; the affected individual attempts to ignore, suppress, or neutralize them. Compulsions are repetitive behaviours or mental acts that the individual feels driven to perform in response to an obsession or according to rigidly applied rules; these are aimed at reducing anxiety or distress. The obsessions or compulsions must be time-consuming, cause significant distress, or impair functioning to meet criteria for OCD. Level of insight and lifetime presence of tics are included as specifiers in the Diagnostic and Statistical Manual of Mental Disorders (American Psychiatric Association, 2013). Children with OCD may not always realize that their worries or behaviours are excessive, viewing rituals as protective acts; nevertheless, a recent international mega-analysis led by our group demonstrated a range of insight in children and adolescents as in adults (Selles, Højgaard et al., 2018). Symptoms that may be more common in children compared to adults include religious and somatic symptoms, "just right" obsessions, compulsions that may involve family members such as parents, and superstitious rituals associated with magical thinking (Kalra & Swedo, 2009). While interventions across the OCD life course clearly improve outcomes and opportunities for affected individuals, the greatest societal and mental health benefits are likely to emerge from interventions that occur in childhood and soon after the onset of the disorder (WHO & CGF, 2014).

Social Determinants of Health and OCD

This section explores familial and social factors influencing OCD symptoms in children. It first examines the epidemiology of the disease with a focus on existing knowledge about geographic and cultural influences on documented prevalence. This is followed by a review of the risk factors for the development of OCD, including environmental factors that have been examined to date. The next sections examine experiences of children and families living with OCD, its long-term impacts on the child's development and function, and familial factors contributing to symptom severity and treatment gains. This is followed by an overview of effective therapies for management of childhood-onset OCD and associated disparities in access to treatment, including social determinants affecting help-seeking behaviours and engagement with mental health care. Finally, practice and research priorities are highlighted with the goal of understanding and modifying the impact of social determinants affecting the long-term function and quality of life of children and families.

General Epidemiology

Most epidemiological studies report OCD prevalence rates between 0.25 and 4 per cent (Douglass et al., 1995; Flament et al., 1988; Heyman et al., 2001), although exact prevalence is affected by the Diagnostic and Statistical Manual of Mental Disorders version used to determine the diagnosis (S.E. Stewart, Hezel et al., 2012). There is no evidence of significant differences in prevalence based on geography (Fogel, 2003). Indeed, epidemiological adult and paediatric studies across multiple international sites suggest that overall OCD prevalence and severity does not differ across ethnic groups or socio-economic strata (Horwath & Weissman, 2000; Medeiros et al., 2017). Data from Canadian epidemiological studies suggest a 2.3 per cent lifetime prevalence (Weissman et al., 1994), similar in males and females, in two groups with mean ages of onset at 9.7 and 21.1 years (De Luca et al., 2011). A more recent population-based health survey by Statistics Canada, which may reflect this disorder's putative under-recognition and under-diagnosis, identified a prevalence of diagnosed OCD of 0.93 per cent (Osland et al., 2018). Health care utilization was more frequent in individuals with diagnosed OCD, but they were also more likely than respondents without OCD to believe they had not received the help they required (Osland et al., 2018). Approximately half of all patients with OCD present before age 15 (Karno et al., 1988). There are three peaks of onset in males, the first pre-puberty at 8 to 10 years, the second in early adulthood between 18 and 22, and the third later in the second decade (Anholt et al., 2013; Geller et al., 1998; Ruscio et al., 2010). In females, peak onset occurs between 10 and 20 years (Ruscio et al., 2010).

It is unclear whether OCD prevalence (as opposed to diagnosed OCD rates) has remained stable over time. A nationwide register-based study in Finland examined sex-specific incidence time trends and characterized sociodemographic risk factors in 3,372 OCD cases compared to 13,372 matched controls (Rintala et al., 2017). Between 1987 and 2001, incidence by age 15 among three cohorts increased from 12.4 to 23.7 /10,000 live born males and 8.5 to 28.0 /10,000 live born females. Seventy-three per cent of the sample with OCD had a co-morbid psychiatric diagnosis; males were more likely to have co-morbid psychotic and developmental disorders, and females to have depressive and anxiety disorders. In this study, higher maternal socio-economic position – as well as well as birth in an urban compared to rural area – was associated with an increased risk of OCD treated in specialist health care. It is important to note that this observed increased risk may be related to increased awareness or higher referral and treatment access rates among families with higher socio-economic status, rather than a true reflection of increasing incidence (Rintala et al., 2017).

OCD Prevalence across Distinct Regions and Cultures

Ethnicity is a social construct referring to shared cultural characteristics and regional identity of a group of individuals (Sheldon & Parker, 1992). Although it does not appear to affect OCD prevalence, ethnic and cultural identity can modify illness narration, patterns of symptoms, and choices of care (Lewis-Fernandez et al., 2014). The impact of cultural identity on

OCD symptoms has received relatively little attention. A recent review of culture in OCD – including studies that incorporate geographic location as a proxy for culture or ethnicity – found similar symptom clusters across studies, consistent with fundamental underlying disease processes (Nicolini et al., 2017). Most data also suggest that religion is similarly not a causal influence in OCD (Nestadt et al., 1998). However, some cultural experiences, including adherence to religious beliefs about the importance of maintaining mental control, may increase the propensity for subclinical obsessive compulsive symptoms (Inozu et al., 2012). In a cross-cultural comparison of OCD symptoms in Turkish and Canadian university students, Turkish participants were more likely to utilize worry and thought suppression as methods of thought control, while Canadian participants tended to use more self-punishment (Yorulmaz et al., 2010). Thus, despite similar prevalence of clinical OCD and similar metacognitive vulnerabilities, some related cognitive processes may vary across cultures or geographies (Yorulmaz et al., 2010). Unfortunately, most existing studies on the topic do not control for differences in education, access to health services, nutrition, and the genetic structure of populations that may differ across ethnic groups (Nicolini et al., 2017).

Because ethnic minorities access fewer mental health services than European Caucasians in Western countries (Wetterneck et al., 2012), demographic information obtained from clinical populations and from health service utilization databases have significant limitations. Barriers to receiving a diagnosis or appropriate treatment may include negative stigma attached to mental health as well as language, socio-economic, and cultural factors. Moreover, OCD often goes undetected in primary care settings (Simonds & Elliott, 2001); Whitaker and colleagues (1990) reported a lifetime prevalence of 1.9 per cent in a non-referred population of US secondary school students, only 25 per cent of whom had seen a mental health professional. There is a need for better understanding of both the epidemiology and barriers to care for OCD in Canadians – and in particular children – of all cultural and geographic backgrounds. Further examination of the impacts of race-based discrimination, victimization, and resiliency factors on access to and experience of care is also needed.

OCD Prevalence and Socio-economic Position

Socio-economic factors, including education and financial status, may affect symptom expression, although no definitive evidence exists regarding causation. Subthreshold OCD symptoms are common and their prevalence may suggest a public health burden beyond that created exclusively by those meeting full diagnostic criteria (Ruscio et al., 2010). For example, in a sample of 7,054 community youth from the Philadelphia Neurodevelopmental Cohort, the prevalence of OCD was 3 per cent but the prevalence of OCD symptoms was up to 38 per cent in non-mental-health service-seeking individuals (Barzilay et al., 2019). This is consistent with a model in which the diagnosis represents the extreme end of continuously distributed traits (Taylor et al., 2018). In this large and racially diverse sample, children with at least one OCD symptom compared to those with none were more likely to be female, non-white, and of lower socio-economic status (Barzilay et al., 2019). Some small studies have also suggested that OCD symptoms among children with a family member who has OCD are associated with socio-economic status. Similarly, in a nationally representative non-clinical sample of 3,570 African American adults, material hardship was associated with most measured symptoms of OCD and fewer years of education was related to greater compulsive symptoms (Williams et al., 2017). Thus, socio-economic differences may be associated with subclinical OCD symptoms in both children and adults, although the direction of the relationship and potential causality are unclear.

OCD in Canadian Indigenous Peoples

In Canada, Indigenous populations comprise First Nations (60.8 per cent), Métis (32.3 per cent), and Inuit (4.2 per cent) peoples (Statistics Canada, 2013b). No studies exist characterizing prevalence of and treatment for OCD in Indigenous populations, although some reports on anxiety disorders may include OCD (as OCD was previously identified as an anxiety disorder). These data provide some insight into common co-morbidities as well as the context in which individuals with OCD may struggle to manage a psychiatric condition.

Using data from the 2002 Canadian Community Health Survey, Caron and Liu (2010) found that Indigenous Canadians over the age of fifteen living off-reserve were more likely to report suffering from psychological distress, mental health disorders, or substance use disorders compared to the general Canadian population. A more recent study of adults living off-reserve identified a high prevalence of self-reported anxiety disorders (Nasreen et al., 2018). High rates of distress were also found in the 2008–10 First Nations Regional Health Survey, in which 50.7 per cent of First Nations adult respondents living on-reserve reported feeling moderately or highly distressed (First Nations Information Governance Centre, 2012). In contrast, findings from a retrospective chart review of 2,375 Indigenous and non-Indigenous patients living in Bella Coola Valley, British Columbia, suggest that depression and anxiety disorder prevalence rates were similar (Thommasen et al., 2005). A Canadian study of urban women accessing social services agencies and shelters also found similarly high lifetime rates of anxiety, depression, and suicide attempts in both Aboriginal and non-Aboriginal populations (Hamdullahpur et al., 2017). However, these studies of specific rural and urban populations with unique risk factors may not be generalizable to other Indigenous populations. Moreover, risk factors for specific disorders may change across the lifespan, underscoring the need for further research aimed at understanding how social determinants, including living conditions and ethnicity, affect the onset and persistence of OCD in Canadian adults and children.

Social Determinants Affecting the Development of OCD Symptoms

Meta-analyses of family studies suggest heritability between 45 to 65 per cent (Mataix-Cols et al., 2013; Nestadt et al., 2000), higher than most other anxiety and mood disorders in youth and higher than in patients with adult-onset illness (Eley et al., 2003). The biology and pathophysiology of childhood-onset OCD – including the role of specific genetic and epigenetic risk factors, infections, and perinatal complications – are discussed in our recent review (Westwell-Roper & Stewart, 2019). Here we briefly comment on social determinants affecting OCD symptoms.

Social and Familial Risk Factors

OCD remains understudied in ethno-racial minority populations in Western countries (Williams & Jahn, 2017). The presence of OCD and the individual, familial, and cultural factors that influence this condition can interfere with healthy development and cause lifelong disability. Ethnic and racial minorities with OCD are under-represented or absent from treatment centres and research studies. While cultural differences in symptomology, low income, reduced access to care, racism, and mental health stigma have been conceptualized as risk factors in African American groups (Williams & Jahn, 2017), definitive evidence is lacking. These factors nevertheless likely affect the experience of the child and family with OCD as well as treatment-seeking behaviours and access to care. Additional family factors are involved in the maintenance and severity of the disorder and may vary among cultural groups; these include family accommodation, conflictual family communication, and parenting styles (Williams & Jahn, 2017). Familial factors that include parental modelling, expressed emotion, parenting style, and family accommodation may be risk factors for persistence of OCD symptoms rather than for the development of the disorder (Chambless et al., 2007; Przeworski et al., 2012; Waters & Barrett, 2000).

Adverse Childhood Experiences

Adverse childhood experiences describe all types of abuse, neglect, and other potentially traumatic events that children under the age of eighteen can experience. As an important determinant of health, they have been linked to risky health behaviours, chronic health conditions, low life potential, and early death (Centers for Disease Control and Prevention [CDCP], 2019a). Adults with untreated OCD report higher rates of exposure to adverse childhood experiences compared to those receiving treatment, despite comparable age, education, age at onset, duration, and severity (Benedetti et al., 2014). This effect is greater in female patients as compared to male patients, suggesting that the interaction of gender with early childhood experiences affects access to psychiatric care or use of medication independent of symptom severity (Benedetti et al., 2014). Several recent studies of adverse childhood experiences in OCD suggest that the association between adverse childhood experiences and OCD symptoms is primarily mediated by co-morbidities, in particular anxiety and mood disorders (Briggs & Price, 2009; Micali et al., 2010; Visser et al., 2014).

The Experience of Living with Childhood-Onset OCD

Children and youth with OCD experience substantial disruptions in social, academic, and interpersonal functioning, with important implications for neurodevelopment. Childhood experiences in turn influence multiple social determinants (see table 3.1). This section reviews the disease course, symptom clusters, co-morbidities, quality of life, and functional outcomes in the context of our existing knowledge about social determinants of health. Their contribution to the life course of children with OCD is summarized in figure 3.1.

Disease Trajectory

Meta-analyses of longitudinal data, including one by our group, suggest that approximately 40 per cent of children have childhood-onset OCD that persists into adulthood, with one-third experiencing moderate to severe symptoms and 20 per cent experiencing subclinical symptoms or partial remission at follow-up (Bloch et al., 2009; Micali et al., 2010; S.E.

Table 3.1. Determinants of Health Affected by OCD Symptoms

Disease-Related Predictor	Impact on Social Determinant of Health[a]	Reference
Presence of Childhood-Onset OCD	Educational attainment	Pérez-Vigil et al., 2018
	Academic achievement (math performance, homework completion)	Negreiros et al., 2018; Piacentini et al., 2003
	Physical health[b] (co-morbidities, including migraines, respiratory diseases, immune-related diseases, infections)	Mataix-Cols et al., 2017; Orlovska et al., 2017; Westwell-Roper et al., 2019; Witthauer et al., 2014
OCD Severity	Role impairment (adults)	Ruscio et al., 2010
	Social, school, family, and occupational functioning (adults and children)	Koran et al., 1996; Piacentini et al., 2003, 2007; Thomsen, 1995
	Marital status (separated or divorced); relationship satisfaction (adults)	Abbey et al., 2007; Subramaniam et al., 2012
	Quality of life in adults (marital status and symptom severity contribute to magnitude of impairment)	Eisen et al., 2006; Subramaniam et al., 2013; Velloso et al., 2018
	Quality of life in children	Storch et al., 2018
Family Accommodation	Overall family function; family occupational impairment	S.E. Stewart, Hu et al., 2017
Co-morbidity Severity	Quality of life in children	Storch et al., 2018

a Outcomes closely linked with a health determinant or measure as defined by WHO or Health Canada (see figure 3.1).
b Factors affecting mental health and specifically persistence of OCD symptoms are discussed in detail in the text and not included in this table.

Stewart, Geller et al., 2004). A major predictor for persistence identified by our study (S.E. Stewart, Geller et al., 2004) and others (Micali et al., 2010) was the duration of illness, which underscores the importance of early recognition and treatment. Symptom persistence has also been associated with the female gender, the absence of a co-morbid tic disorder, the presence of prominent hoarding symptoms, an earlier age at childhood assessment, a later age of onset, more severe OCD symptoms, and co-morbid oppositional defiant disorder (Bloch et al., 2009). Other factors that contribute to a more disabling course include early co-morbid major depressive disorder, parental psychopathology, and a poor response to medication (Denys et al., 2003; Leonard et al., 1992;

Figure 3.1. Social determinants of health affecting the course and management of OCD. Health determinants (red boxes, as defined by Health Canada, 2019) modify disease onset, symptom content and associated distress, early intervention, and response to treatment. Socio-economic and familial factors provide a backdrop against which interactions with the health care system shape the child's experiences and, ultimately, multiple social and health-related outcomes through adolescence and beyond

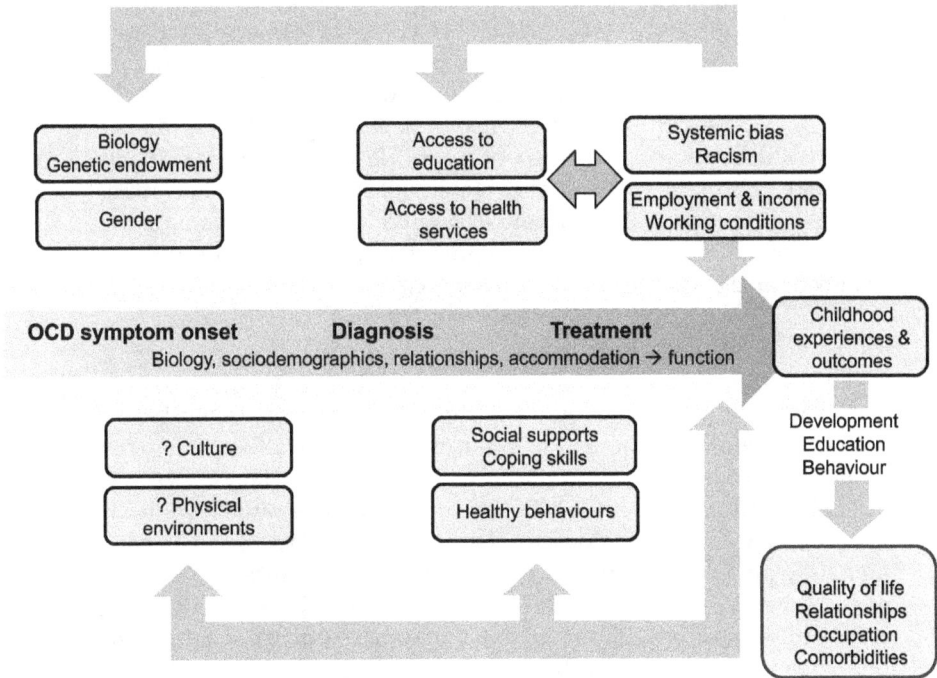

Shetti et al., 2005; Skoog & Skoog, 1999). Factors that may contribute to a more benign OCD course include the presence of a precipitating event, episodic symptoms, and good social and occupational adjustment (Denys et al., 2003; Sadock & Sadock, 2002). Because delays in treatment also predict persistence, it is important to understand the sociocultural factors affecting access to psychiatric care.

OCD Symptoms

Overlapping groups or "symptom dimensions" are generally stable throughout development and include symmetry or perfectionism (symmetry obsessions and repeating, ordering, and counting compulsions), guilt or forbidden thoughts (violent, sexual, religious, and somatic obsessions and checking compulsions), and cleaning (contamination obsessions and cleaning compulsions), as well as hoarding (S.E. Stewart, Rosário et al., 2008). Other common compulsions include reassurance-seeking, counting, praying, and mental rituals. A recent international mega-analysis led by our group found that 88.9 per cent of children had fair to excellent insight into these symptoms, 9.7 per cent had poor insight, and only 1.4 per cent had insight in the absent/delusional category (Selles, Højgaard et al., 2018). Worse insight was associated with increased distress and avoidance and decreased symptom resistance (Selles, Højgaard et al., 2018). Symptom dimensions appear to be relatively stable across cultures and geographies, although their prevalence may vary with context and country of origin (Li et al., 2009; Matsunaga et al., 2008; Yorulmaz et al., 2010). Table 3.2 summarizes associations identified in selected studies by ourselves and others that examine the influence of culture, race, socio-economic status, and other social determinants of health on OCD-related outcomes.

Sleep

Sleep plays a fundamental role in the physical, emotional, and behavioural health and development of children (Dahl, 2007). Poor sleep has also been associated with multiple social and economic factors (Grandner et al., 2015). A recent study by our group demonstrated a clinically relevant sleep disturbance in 70 per cent of children with OCD compared to 15 per cent of healthy controls, particularly increased wakening, delayed subsequent sleep, and poorer sleep hygiene (Jaspers-Fayer et al., 2018). Children with OCD and insomnia may have poorer general functioning compared to those without sleep disturbances, and remain more severely affected after treatment (Sevilla-Cermeño et al., 2019). Sleep disturbance therefore represents an important vulnerability tied to multiple social determinants of health and requires careful consideration in the assessment and treatment of this disorder.

Suicide

An elevated risk of suicide attempts and death by suicide exists across all relatives of children and adults with OCD, increasing in proportion to the degree of genetic relatedness (Sidorchuk et al., 2019). Familial co-aggregation of OCD and suicide attempts is explained by additive genetic factors (60 per cent) as well as the non-shared environment (40 per cent), pointing to combined social and biological risk factors that

Table 3.2. Aspects of OCD Affected by Specific Social Determinants of Health

Predictor[a]	OCD-Related Measure	Effect	Reference[b]
Gender	Lifetime prevalence	None	S.E. Stewart, Negreiros et al., 2016
	Co-morbidity profile	More psychotic and developmental disorders in males, depressive and anxiety disorders in females	Rintala et al., 2017
Socio-economic Status (SES)	Treatment by specialist	Increased OCD prevalence with higher SES based on treatment received in specialist care	Rintala et al., 2017
	Prevalence	None	Alvarenga et al., 2016; Douglass et al., 1995; Horwath & Weissman, 2000; Medeiros et al., 2017
Income	Global and financial burden of OCD	Increased global and financial burden of OCD and increased disturbance in family routine and leisure activities with lower income	Vikas et al., 2011
	General and psychological QOL	Greater financial burden associated with lower QOL	Grover & Dutt, 2011
Rural Residence	Financial burden of OCD	Greater financial burden associated with rural vs. urban residence	Vikas et al., 2011
Parental Education	Prevalence	None	Douglass et al., 1995
	Symptom recognition	Adults with higher education better able to recognize symptoms as OCD	Chong et al., 2016

(*Continued*)

Table 3.2. (Continued)

Predictor[a]	OCD-Related Measure	Effect	Reference[b]
Culture, Ethnicity, Geography, or Religion	Prevalence	None	Horwath & Weissman, 2000; Medeiros et al., 2017; Nestadt et al., 1998
	Symptom attribution	Causal attributions for symptoms vary among Americans, Europeans, and Asians	Yang et al., 2018
	Help-seeking	Minority status (UK) associated with more perceived barriers to care and less help-seeking	Fernández de la Cruz et al., 2016
	Treatment	Minority status (North America) associated with under-representation in mental health services; less likely to receive treatment	Fernandez de la Cruz et al., 2015; Grace et al., 2016; Himle et al., 2008
	Treatment outcomes	None	Thompson-Hollands et al., 2014
	Symptom dimensions/content	Some studies suggest consistent symptom dimensions; others point to differences in symptom content or metacognitive processes	Li et al., 2009; Matsunaga et al., 2008; Williams, Elstein et al., 2012; Yorulmaz et al., 2010
	Representation in clinical trials and genome-wide association studies	Minority status in North America associated with under-representation in clinical trials and genetics studies	S.E.Stewart, Yu et al., 2013; Wetterneck et al., 2012; Williams et al., 2010
Adverse childhood experience (ACE)	Symptom severity	None	Visser et al., 2014
	Co-morbidity	ACE's associated with co-morbid affective disorders, substance use disorders, and eating disorders	Briggs & Price, 2009; Visser et al., 2014
	Treatment	ACE's associated with self-reported untreated symptoms in females	Benedetti et al., 2014

Predictor[a]	OCD-Related Measure	Effect	Reference[b]
Stressful life event (SLE)	Severity	History of at least one traumatic event associated with increased severity	Cromer et al., 2007
	Symptom content	Higher rates of obsessions/checking and symmetry/ordering in patients with OCD and a history of SLE	Cromer et al., 2007
Family communication	Prevalence	Higher expressed emotion in mothers of children with vs. without OCD; specific to child with OCD vs. sibling	Hibbs et al., 1993; Przeworski et al., 2012
Family accommodation; family burden	Treatment outcome	Remission associated with lower levels of family accommodation	Cherian et al., 2014

a Predictor related to social determinant of health as defined by the WHO or Health Canada (figure 3.1).
b Selected references only as discussed in text.

may allow targeting of high-risk groups for prevention and treatment (Sidorchuk et al., 2019). In children with OCD, suicidal ideation is significantly related to clinician-rated depressive symptoms, age, child-rated impairment and anxiety symptoms, symmetry, sexuality/religiosity and miscellaneous symptom dimensions (Storch et al., 2015). More work is needed to determine how social determinants modify the risk of suicidal ideation or attempts in children with OCD. For example, rates of youth suicide in Indigenous children in Canada far dramatically exceed the national average (Greenwood & de Leeuw, 2012), but there are no existing studies addressing the interaction among race/ethnicity, suicide risk, and OCD. This interaction would need to explore not only the social determinants of heath, such as income, employment and education, but also the more distal determinants that include racism (Paradies et al., 2013) and racist colonialist policies such as residential schools (Brave Heart, 2011; TRCC, 2015). Further, suicide is a complex phenomenon, and for First Nations youth in British Columbia, it has been linked to a variety of community-level factors (Chandler & Lalonde, 1998), necessitating a sophisticated strengths-based analysis to better elucidate these interactions.

Co-morbidities

Up to 80 per cent of children and adolescents with OCD have one or more co-morbid psychiatric conditions, pointing to a clustering of vulnerabilities. Close to half meet criteria for a co-morbid anxiety or depressive disorder. The most common co-morbidities include major depressive disorder, attention deficit hyperactivity disorder, oppositional defiant disorder, anxiety disorders, enuresis, and speech and language disorders (Geller et al., 2000). Tics occur in 10–40 per cent of patients with childhood-onset OCD (Leckman et al., 2011). The presence of co-morbidities may affect an appropriate treatment strategy (Brauer et al., 2011) as well as treatment response (Storch et al., 2008).

Psychiatric disorders also impact physical health. While limited data addressing the prevalence of medical co-morbidities exists for childhood-onset OCD, multiple conditions, including migraines and respiratory diseases, are more common among adults with OCD (Witthauer et al., 2014). Some of these co-morbidities are more common among those with low household income or food insecurity (Nagata et al., 2019), which might be expected in OCD as well. Our group recently described self-reported rates of immune-related conditions among participants with childhood-onset OCD in the Obsessive Compulsive Disorder Collaborative Genetics Association Study (Westwell-Roper et al., 2019). Comparison with population rates suggested higher than expected prevalence of streptococcal-related and other immune-related diseases, consistent with epidemiological studies in adults noting familial clustering (Mataix-Cols et al., 2017). An improved understanding of shared genetic and environmental risks for co-morbid medical conditions – in addition to the effects of medical co-morbidities on OCD symptom content – may pave the way for further interventional trials and facilitate collaborative multidisciplinary care for children affected by multiple physical and psychiatric conditions.

Functional Implications

Close to half of children and adolescents with OCD suffer notable illness-related impairments in social, school, and family functioning (Piacentini et al., 2003). These impairments appear to be related to frequent participation in rituals and associated distress. More severe or long-standing illness is associated with increased levels of functional impairment (Piacentini et al., 2007). OCD is often associated with difficulties in interpersonal relationships, with even subclinical OCD symptoms linked to impairments in social function (Abbey et al., 2007). Some studies have found that marital status (divorced or separated) is associated with OCD in adults, emphasizing the potential long-term impact of persistent childhood-onset OCD on relationships (Palardy et al., 2018; Subramaniam et al., 2012). Severity of obsessions is negatively correlated with intimacy, relationship satisfaction, and self-disclosure, even after controlling for depressive symptoms (Abbey et al., 2007). These factors have the potential to influence an individual's social supports, further contributing to social determinants of health later in life.

Quality of Life

Quality of life is linked to an individual's perceived physical and mental health and their correlates, including health risks and conditions, function, social support, and socio-economic position (CDCP, 2019b). In children, greater parental education has a positive impact on physical well-being, psychological well-being, moods and emotions, and bullying (von Rueden et al., 2006). In children with OCD, quality of life is further affected by symptom severity and impairment (Storch et al., 2018). Most studies suggest that OCD symptom severity and co-morbid major depressive disorder or depressive symptoms are predictors of decreased quality of life, with numerous reports showing this association across multiple domains (Velloso et al., 2018). Few studies have measured quality of life and its response to treatment in children with OCD, although the Pediatric Quality of Life Enjoyment and Satisfaction Questionnaire shows good reliability and validity in adolescents (Wellen et al., 2017). Scores using this tool are strongly associated with the presence of co-morbid major depressive disorder, suggesting that addressing co-morbid conditions is an important component of intensive treatment (Zaboski et al., 2019). Treatment, including family-focused cognitive behavioural therapy, also leads to improvements in parent-reported quality of life measures (Storch et al., 2018). There is a need for studies assessing quality of life in both clinical and community samples of adequate size to examine additional sociodemographic correlates (Subramaniam et al., 2013).

Academic Skills

Academic outcomes in early adolescence are affected by gender, race (likely primarily as a risk factor for the experience of racism), home intellectual materials, emotional control, and family involvement (Li et al., 2017). Mental health is also an important predictor of academic performance in children (Murphy et al., 2015). Students with OCD report having difficulty concentrating on school work and homework completion (Piacentini et al., 2003). A recent study by our group identified significantly poorer performance in math calculation in patients with childhood-onset OCD compared to healthy controls (Negreiros et al., 2018), and we have also observed subtle deficits affecting planning (Jaspers-Fayer et al., 2017; Kim et al., 2019; S.E. Stewart, Negreiros et al., 2016). Underperformance on tasks assessing processing speed may similarly be important in clinical and school settings (Geller et al., 2018). Academic skills in childhood may in turn be linked to educational attainment and occupational function later in life, suggesting one mechanism by which childhood-onset OCD is not only influenced by but also affects social determinants of health. Childhood-onset OCD is associated with a pervasive decrease in educational attainment, as demonstrated by a recent Swedish birth cohort study (Pérez-Vigil et al., 2018). Further studies of academic skills may help to identify potential strategies for enhancing academic performance and identifying children who can benefit most.

Role and Experience of Family in Childhood-Onset OCD

The accumulation of familial adversity factors – for example, socioeconomic risk or parent psychiatric history – increases the risk for general paediatric psychopathology (Wiik et al., 2011). Children experience culture, social norms, social policies, and political systems through their incorporation and interpretation by the family (Deatrick, 2017). Caregivers play a key role in modifying risks of the external environment for the child, but are also vulnerable themselves; indeed, parents of OCD-affected children represent an underserved population (Lebowitz, 2017). We have found that Mindfulness Skills-Based Intervention significantly helped parents to tolerate their child's distress (a key component in limiting detrimental OCD accommodation) in comparison to waitlist control conditions (Belschner et al., 2020). In general, parents are most likely to report lack of partnerships with health care providers if their children have functional limitations, are from ethnic or racial minorities, have low incomes, do not have health insurance, and have limited English language skills in English-speaking countries (Deatrick, 2017). In a recent study, we found that parents of Asian compared to Caucasian OCD-affected youth reported lower likelihood of OCD treatment, despite similar treatment recommendation patterns (Wang et al., 2020). The consequences for children of limited engagement with health care providers may include more missed school days, fewer referrals for services, unmet medical needs, and less satisfaction with the care they receive (Deatrick, 2017). This section reviews the impact of OCD on the family, as well as family behaviours that may perpetuate OCD symptoms and the critical role of the family in treatment.

Impact of OCD on the Family

The impact of OCD on family members has been well documented, with the child's OCD symptoms impairing marital, social, school and occupational functioning (Cooper, 1996; Piacentini et al., 2003; Stengler-Wenzke et al., 2006; Vikas et al., 2011). The OCD Family Functioning Scale was developed by S.E. Stewart to explore the context, extent, and perspectives of functional impairment in families affected by OCD (S.E. Stewart, Hu et al., 2011). In a multisite study of family functioning impairment, our team found that 50 per cent of mothers, 30 per cent of fathers, and 70 per cent of youth reported daily occupational/school impacts (M. Stewart, Hu et al., 2017). Most youth and their parents reported often or always feeling stressed/anxious or frustrated/angry. Commonly disrupted routines related to bedtime, morning, family events, mealtimes, and work/school (M. Stewart, Hu et al., 2017). Caregivers and relatives of patients with OCD consistently report lower quality of life, regardless of geographic location or cultural context (Grover & Dutt, 2011; Stengler-Wenzke et al., 2006; Vikas et al., 2011). Multiple sociodemographic factors may affect both objective and perceived family burden: although in samples with high overall socio-economic status this is not necessarily the case (Farmer et al., 2018). A study of families in North West India revealed a negative correlation between income and multiple measures of family burden (Vikas et al., 2011). Residence in a rural location had a significant correlation with financial burden, suggesting that the impact of OCD on the family may be modified by geography and access to appropriate care.

Family Accommodation

The impairment experienced by family members is partially a consequence of parental involvement in their child's OCD symptoms (Calvocoressi et al., 1995; Storch et al., 2007; Wu et al., 2016). Family accommodation refers to ways in which family members take part in the performance of rituals, facilitate avoidance of anxiety-provoking situations, or modify routine. We have found that family accommodation is common and occurs on a daily basis in many families, with most common behaviours including reassurance and waiting for ritual completion (S.E. Stewart, Beresin et al., 2008). This study, as well as a recent meta-analysis, emphasized the strong link between family accommodation and OCD symptom severity (S.E. Stewart, Beresin et al., 2008; Strauss et al., 2015). Co-morbid anxiety disorders may moderate this relationship (Wu et al., 2019).

Family members report negative feelings when assisting in rituals or modifying their routines because of OCD. On the other hand, they also report distress when refusing to assist in rituals due to frustration expressed by their OCD-affected relatives (Amir et al., 2000). Not engaging in a child's OCD rituals can be particularly distressing for the parent, especially when the child responds with rage (Storch et al., 2012) or coercive behaviours (Lebowitz et al., 2011). However, the resulting accommodation inadvertently worsens the child's OCD (Peris et al., 2012; Wu et al., 2016). Accordingly, several studies have shown that reducing family accommodation results in better treatment outcomes for OCD-affected children (Amir et al., 2000; Garcia et al., 2010; Strauss et al., 2015). Our group has also found that parents' distress tolerance – a positive outcome predictor in childhood-onset OCD (Freeman et al., 2008; Peris & Miklowitz, 2015; Selles, Franklin, et al., 2018) – improves significantly over the course of family-focused cognitive behavioural therapy. Sociodemographic variables have not been associated with family accommodation (Wu et al., 2019), although additional appropriately powered studies to understand better how social determinants of health affect family accommodation and distress are needed.

Role of Family in OCD Treatment

Children with OCD benefit from treatment tailored to their developmental needs and family context (Freeman et al., 2008). A meta-analysis of forty-eight general child psychotherapy outcome studies suggested that including parents in the psychotherapeutic treatment adds benefits beyond individual child therapies (Dowell & Ogles, 2010). Indeed, nearly all programs for childhood-onset OCD include some degree of parent-involvement as demonstrated by our group and others (Anderson et al., 2015; Lebowitz & Shimshoni, 2018; Selles, Belschner et al., 2018). The modality of choice for paediatric OCD is cognitive behavioural therapy, specifically utilizing exposure and response prevention, in which children learn to gradually expose themselves to their OCD-related fears and obsessions while resisting engagement in rituals and avoidant behaviours (Freeman et al., 2018; Watson & Rees, 2008). Our research team recently demonstrated that a group-and-family-based cognitive behavioural therapy program significantly improves a wide range of domains for youth and families (Selles, Belschner et al., 2018). Other studies have similarly demonstrated a large overall effect on OCD symptoms and global functioning with family-inclusive treatment, particularly with approaches targeting family accommodation (Thompson-Hollands et al., 2014). Families with lower levels of parental blame and family conflict and higher levels of family cohesion at baseline may be more likely to have a child who responds to treatment (Peris et al., 2012). Based on existing studies, there appears to be no significant effect of ethnicity or age group on treatment success (Thompson-Hollands et al., 2014).

Although there is a clear need for support for parents of OCD-affected children (Stengler-Wenzke et al., 2006; S.E. Stewart, Hu et al., 2017), few interventions are specifically aimed at helping them cope with their own and their child's emotional distress (Lebowitz, 2017). Recent work by our group has shown promising effects of a mindfulness-based intervention for parents on their tolerance of their children's distress. Other forms of treatment involving the family include positive family interaction therapy (Belschner et al., 2020), which may help reduce OCD symptom severity and impairment and improve family functioning (Peris et al., 2017).

Genetic counselling may also provide a mechanism to assist parents in understanding and coping with their child's OCD, although access to such expertise is limited. Our research team has conducted qualitative semi-structured telephone interviews with parents of children diagnosed with OCD to explore participants' experiences with their child's illness, causal attributions, and perceptions of two genetic counselling vignettes (Andrighetti et al., 2016). The process by which parents adapted to their child's illness involved conceptualizing the meaning of OCD, navigating its impact on the family, and developing management strategies. Adaptation was affected by stigma, family history of mental illness, and the child's symptoms. Parents perceived genetic counselling as empowering and reported it helped to alleviate guilt and blame. It also positively impacted treatment orientation (Andrighetti et al., 2016), a potentially critical outcome given multiple barriers to seeking and accessing care.

Interventions and Inequities in Childhood-Onset OCD

Despite the availability of effective treatments, the duration of untreated illness in OCD is high and associated with considerable suffering for children and their families. A recent consensus statement by an international group of clinicians describes the negative impacts associated with treatment delays and the importance of early intervention (Fineberg et al., 2019). The authors conclude that there is a global unmet need for early intervention services for OCD-related disorders to reduce unnecessary suffering and costly disability associated with undertreatment. This section reviews the general approach to treatment of childhood-onset

OCD, factors affecting access to treatment, and other barriers to care that may result from and also contribute to health inequities.

General Treatment Approach

The two first-line, evidence-based treatment approaches for management of paediatric OCD are cognitive behavioural therapy and serotonin reuptake inhibitor medications, including both selective serotonin reuptake inhibitors and clomipramine. For further discussion of these and other emerging treatments for childhood-onset OCD, we refer the reader to our recent review (Westwell-Roper & Stewart, 2019). In brief, cognitive behavioural therapy is typically the initial treatment of choice for children with mild to moderate OCD, in combination with serotonin reuptake inhibitors for moderate to severe cases (Geller & March, 2012; Pediatric OCD Treatment Study Team, 2004). For cases in which potential medication side effects outweigh benefits, including those with mild illness, an initial trial of cognitive behavioural therapy alone may be more effective than medication (Ivarsson et al., 2015). Multiple factors have been associated with treatment outcomes, largely related to features of the disorder and family's response (Chu et al., 2015; Garcia et al., 2010; Torp et al., 2015). There is no evidence to date that sociodemographic factors or stressful life events at onset predict treatment response (Alemany-Navarro et al., 2019). However, it is unclear how effective empirically validated treatments may be for minority groups with under-representation in North American trials. Of forty randomized controlled trials that included patients with OCD in the United States and Canada from 1989 to 2009, only twenty-one trials provided ethnic/racial information and close to 92 per cent of participants were Caucasian (Williams et al., 2010). Some ethnic minorities have been excluded. The lack of diversity in existing trials has led funding agencies to require investigators to specifically address this issue; however, barriers to trial participation are complex and not fully understood.

For severe, refractory cases of childhood-onset OCD, including those with significant co-morbidities, intensive residential treatment with up to twenty-seven hours per week of exposure and response prevention may be effective (Leonard et al., 2016). The first long-term follow-up study of intensive residential treatment in adults with OCD, led by S.E. Stewart, found maintenance of treatment gains up to six months post-discharge (S.E. Stewart, Stack et al., 2009). Those who relapsed were more likely to live alone following discharge, underscoring a potential association with lack of social support, or alternatively relationship impairment associated with other disease-related factors (S.E. Stewart, Stack et al., 2009).

In Canada, there are no residential treatment facilities available for children or youth and only one for adults; those referred for treatment out-of-country may receive financial coverage through provincial health plans, however with the potential to cause significant financial and social burden for the family. Ironically, cognitive behavioural therapy in the community – which should be tried before impairment is so severe as to require residential treatment – is not covered by provincial health plans when offered by private therapists. Moreover, it is often difficult to access outside of overstretched tertiary programs or mental health teams, and there are significant financial barriers for many families.

Availability of Cognitive Behavioural Therapy

Cognitive behavioural therapy for paediatric OCD as delivered in clinical trials is a short-term treatment, usually between twelve and twenty weekly sessions. In an open, uncontrolled study of family-based cognitive behavioural therapy in eighty-five OCD-affected children/teens between the ages of eight and eighteen (recently completed by our group), treatment was associated with significant reductions in OCD severity, youth and parent-rated functional impairment, coercive/disruptive behaviours, family accommodation, and family functioning (Selles, Belschner et al., 2018). Greater homework success predicted symptom improvement. While exposure and response prevention is part of most programs with the best supporting evidence, therapists in the community report using exposure rarely compared with other approaches (Reid et al., 2018). Improvements in access to cognitive behavioural therapy and exposure and response prevention may require increased training opportunities for therapists, in addition to public funding to reduce inequitable access to this gold-standard treatment.

Barriers to Care

Increasing the effective dissemination of existing treatments is a major priority in efforts to reduce the global burden associated with under-treatment of OCD (Fineberg et al., 2019). Common barriers to seeking treatment include shame about the symptoms or about asking for treatment, not knowing where to find help, or inconveniences associated with treatment (García-Soriano et al., 2014). Cost, lack of insurance coverage, and doubt that treatment would be effective are also commonly endorsed barriers (Marques et al., 2010). Barriers to parent involvement in a child's treatment include feeling blamed, judged, unsupported, or generally dissatisfied with health care services (Baker-Ericzen et al.,

2013). Symptom fluctuation may also be a contributing factor to longer duration of untreated illness (Poyraz et al., 2015).

Mental health literacy – a component of which is recognition of symptoms as part of a mental illness – is an important mediating factor in help-seeking behaviour. A nationwide population-based study in Singapore identified OCD among the least recognized psychiatric disorders; younger age and higher education levels were associated with better recognition (Chong et al., 2016). Even among health care professionals, OCD often goes undetected in primary care settings (Simonds & Elliott, 2001; Whitaker et al., 1990). Sociodemographic characteristics influencing mental health literacy need to be considered in planning appropriate education and intervention strategies.

Data from the 1996 US National Anxiety Disorders Screening Day involving 14,860 Americans suggested that individuals with minority racial status were less likely to seek care (Goodwin et al., 2002). Differences in treatment uptake among ethnic groups result from a complex interplay of language barriers, cultural beliefs, mental illness stigma, financial resources, and social resources. With respect to causal attributions, an exploratory study of eighty-nine patients ages fifteen and over in a tertiary hospital in Northern India showed that almost 60 per cent of patients attributed their illness to a supernatural cause. Only two-thirds sought initial care from a psychiatrist, while others sought care from faith healers (Grover et al., 2014). A survey of 428 individuals from thirteen countries also pointed to differences in symptom attribution. Compared to individuals in the United States and Western Europe, participants in East Asia had a more negative view, blaming the person with OCD, and recommending against seeking help from others (Yang et al., 2018). Such beliefs about the cause of symptoms are likely to impact parents' perceptions of their children's illness as well.

Beliefs about the potential benefits of treatment may also vary among cultural groups, particularly in more marginalized and vulnerable populations. A UK study exploring attitudes towards treatment in a group of 293 parents recruited from the general population – comprising White British, Black African, Black Caribbean, and Indian groups with no differences in sociodemographic factors or family history of OCD – found that White British parents perceived that OCD-related difficulties depicted in a text vignette would have more of a negative impact on their children and that treatment would be more helpful, compared to the ethnic minorities (Fernández de la Cruz et al., 2016). Ethnic minorities were more prone to say that they would seek help from their religious communities. Black African parents favoured no help seeking and perceived more treatment barriers (Fernández de la Cruz et al., 2016).

The majority of North American data on ethnicity and OCD treatment are based on small studies of African Americans. For example, the modified Barriers to Treatment Participation Scale and the Barriers to Treatment Questionnaire were completed by seventy-one African American adults and compared to an internet sample of 108 European Americans (Williams, Domanico et al., 2012). Overall, participants identified seven major barriers, including the cost of treatment, stigma, fears of therapy, believing that the clinician will be unable to help, perceiving no need for treatment, and treatment logistics (being too busy or treatment being too inconvenient). Age, gender, income, education, insurance status, and ethnicity affected several scale components. Concerns about cost were significantly greater for those without insurance compared to those with public or private plans, and barriers unique to the African American group included not knowing where to find help and concerns about discrimination (Williams, Domanico et al., 2012).

There are no Canadian data on the proportion of children with OCD receiving treatment, or on perceived barriers to access by families. In adults, a cross-sectional follow-up survey to the 2013 Canadian Community Health Survey found the majority (81.8 per cent) of Canadians with a mood and/or an anxiety disorder diagnosis reported that they were taking medications or had received treatment. Receiving treatment was significantly associated with older age; higher household income; living in the Atlantic region or Quebec versus Ontario; and having concurrent disorders or mood disorders only (O'Donnell et al., 2017). In a survey of ethnoculturally diverse Ontarians, mental health service use was found to be significantly lower in Asian and Black Canadians, but not Indigenous peoples, when compared to Caucasian participants (Grace et al., 2016). This study pointed to a high burden of psychosocial stressors among ethnocultural minorities who access fewer available mental health services (Grace et al., 2016). More research is needed to characterize factors leading to treatment delays and barriers in Canadian children.

Social Determinants of Mental Health: Implications for Practice, Programs, and Policy

Targeting Social Inequities to Improve Child and Youth Mental Health in Canada

Policy solutions must keep in mind the critical role of a child's family environment and focus on alleviating known contributors to poor mental health outcomes, including adverse childhood experiences, socio-economic deprivation, parental substance use, parental mental health, and systemic racism (Houtepen et al., 2020; Zilanawala et al., 2019). To this end, the International Society for Social Paediatrics and Child Health has highlighted specific actions aimed at strengthening individuals and communities, improving living and working conditions, and promoting healthy macro-policies (Spencer et al., 2019). Youth, families, and researchers must be included in planning, implementing, and evaluating changes made at the individual, community, and systems levels. Inequities specifically affecting minority, immigrant, and Indigenous populations underscore the need for a framework of cultural humility and safety (Linton et al., 2019).

Multiple proposed initiatives to address gaps in children's mental health services arose from analyses of data from the 2014 Child Health Study. These include ensuring coherent policy leadership, making comprehensive children's mental health plans that include effective interventions, using innovative service approaches to improve access, addressing avoidable childhood adversity, and ensuring dedicated children's mental health budgets (Waddell et al., 2019). Addressing adversity includes initiatives to reduce family income disparity and unsafe neighbourhoods and broadening children's mental health planning to include housing, recreation, and justice sectors (Waddell et al., 2019).

Transitions through school involve multiple developmental negotiations and represent critical periods of vulnerability for children with mental illness affected by poverty (Tilleczek et al., 2014). In 2015, the Mental Health Commission of Canada published a report detailing steps forward in building a responsive mental health and addictions system for emerging adults (Carver et al., 2015). It argues that our current approaches are substantially limited – both for those transitioning from child to adult services and for those requiring services for the first time – and offers a framework for bettering these practices in Canada, together with proposed actions at the provincial and national levels (Carver et al., 2015). Similarly, Abidi and colleagues examined the lack of coordination between child and adolescent mental health systems and adult mental health systems in Canada leading to disruption of care during this transition period (Abidi, 2017). They advocate for program development for youth with mental illness that does not use age to determine access or readiness for transition.

Stigma is also a major driver of health inequities that can be addressed at the public health level (Tam, 2019). For example, youth from Northern Ontario communities have highlighted stigma as a major barrier – in addition to lack of motivation, long wait-lists, and transportation challenges – to accessing treatment and services for substance use disorders (C. Russell et al., 2019). The 2019 Chief Public Health Officer's Report on the State of Public Health in Canada outlines strategies for building on multiculturalism while at the same time recognizing racism, homophobia, transphobia, and other stigmas related to social identities (Tam, 2019). It emphasizes the need across the health system to stop the use of dehumanizing language, examine assumptions, and implement policies and education programs, while also measuring progress towards stigma elimination.

Focusing on Social Determinants of Health Affecting Childhood-Onset Mental Health Conditions

Lower rates of mental health service use among first-generation immigrant adolescents highlight the need to identify and address barriers to recognition and treatment among children and adolescents from immigrant and racial/ethnic minority backgrounds (Georgiades et al., 2018). However, different profiles of social risk factors may be determined by an individual's culture of origin. In Canadian South Asian immigrant populations, female gender, having no children under the age of twelve, food insecurity, poor-to-fair self-rated health status, being a current smoker, and immigrating to Canada as a child or teen were associated with greater risk of negative mental health outcomes; while unemployment, lack of a regular medical doctor, and limited physical activity were associated with greater risk for South Asian Canadian-born populations (Islam et al., 2014). Other predictors of better mental health among Canadian immigrants include older age, higher income, a better sense of community belonging, and being employed. Although similar Canadian data do not exist for childhood mental disorders such as OCD, these findings emphasize the need to attend to socio-economic determinants – including low income, unemployment, and a poor sense of community belonging – across all population groups (Salami, Yaskina et al., 2017). First steps include characterizing potential risk factors and clinical characteristics among patients and families receiving treatment for childhood-onset OCD. For example, we have recently undertaken a study of clinical characteristics and self-reported race/ethnicity of families attending the BC Children's Hospital Provincial OCD Program (Wang et al., 2020). Comparison of data from clinical and community populations may help to identify profiles of families who are under-represented in clinical care. Given much poorer mental health outcomes compared to the rest of the population, Canadian Indigenous youth are an important priority.

Addressing Social Risks in Mental Health Care

Work at the interface of neuroscience, medicine, public health, and public policy is required to address the social determinants affecting the trajectory of children with mental disorders such as OCD. The WHO *Global Plan of Action on Social Determinants of Health* identifies five goals in taking action against health inequities: enhancing health policies and decision-making; widening participation in policymaking and implementation; improving health care and services; strengthening international cooperation; and monitoring impact and progress (WHO & CGF, 2014). While multiple interventions have been shown to improve some aspects of prenatal, postnatal, family, physical, and social environments for young children, sustainable effects are difficult to achieve (Moore et al., 2015). Reducing inequities during early childhood requires a multifaceted approach that incorporates policies to improve access to quality social services, facilitate secure and flexible workplaces for parents, deliver inclusive and evidence-based therapies, encourage strengthening of community networks, and provide timely information and support to parents (Moore et al., 2015).

Among practitioners and service providers, questions about whether changes to care are needed based on a patient's social risk factors and when such risks should be prioritized in care delivery are often met with no clear consensus (Shields-Zeeman et al., 2019). Approaches include tailoring management plans to reduce the effects of social or economic adversity ("social risk-informed care") or incorporating knowledge of risk factors more directly by connecting patients with services that help reduce social risks ("social risk-targeted care") (Shields-Zeeman et al., 2019). Suggestions for overcoming treatment barriers have included increasing community education to encourage help-seeking behaviours (García-Soriano et al., 2014), development of more affordable and accessible treatment options, and increasing cultural competence among mental health providers (Williams et al., 2012). In children, this requires careful coordination between clinicians and families as well as school personnel.

Improving Access to Services

There is an unmet need for cognitive behavioural therapy in most low- and middle-income countries, and – within North America – outside of tertiary care centres. Various models for training additional practitioners have been proposed, including training and supervision by a small number of highly trained staff to front-line non-specialist staff (Beck et al., 2016).

To illustrate, the Canadian Institute for Obsessive Compulsive Disorders Accreditation Task Force has a mandate to establish specialty OCD certification/accreditation standards and competencies. Its goal is to improve access to evidence-based clinical care for both children and adults with OCD (Sookman & Fineberg, 2015). Across Canada, limited access to psychotherapy in the public health system has disadvantaged those from low-income households unable to obtain more rapid access through private providers. In 2018, the Mental Health Commission of Canada reviewed lessons learned from implementation of psychotherapy programs in the UK and Australia, offering several policy considerations for removing financial barriers that limit access to psychotherapies in Canada (Mental Health Commission of Canada [MHCC], 2018). They recommend universal approaches – either insurance- or grant-based – combined with targeted programming to promote equitable uptake and clear equity goals.

Telephone cognitive behavioural therapy has also been proposed as a potentially cost-effective method to improve access to treatment for childhood-onset OCD. A trial comparing telephone cognitive behavioural therapy to face-to-face cognitive behavioural therapy in seventy-two individuals aged eleven to eighteen found no significant differences in quality-adjusted life years or OCD symptom severity between groups. The authors concluded that telephone cognitive behavioural therapy should be considered a clinically non-inferior alternative, when access to standard clinic-based cognitive behavioural therapy is limited or if preferred by patients (Tie et al., 2019). Along similar lines, a research trial comparing video teleconference-delivered family cognitive behavioural therapy versus clinic-based family cognitive behavioural therapy in twenty-two children aged four to eight with OCD found no significant difference in treatment retention, engagement, symptom trajectories, or family accommodation (Comer et al., 2017).

New technologies are also a potential vehicle to address the challenges faced by traditional cognitive behavioural therapy. For example, therapist-guided internet-delivered cognitive behavioural therapy programs for children (Aspvall et al., 2018) and adolescents (Lenhard et al., 2017) have led to significant improvement in OCD symptoms following treatment; these results were maintained at three-month follow-up (Aspvall et al., 2018; Lenhard et al., 2017). Finally, mental health apps are a potential modality to extend the reach of mental health care beyond the clinic, but data supporting their efficacy in OCD is limited (Van Ameringen et al., 2017). Both telephone and online delivered programs offer potential access to services for childhood mental health disorders and in many areas accessibility has recently increased in the context of the COVID-19 pandemic.

Priorities for Further Research

Multiple social determinants likely affect the experience of the affected child and family, including their levels of distress and function. There is some evidence for differential effects of social determinants on members of different populations, and these require further elucidation. Efforts to develop a more comprehensive understanding of the optimal time and dosage of certain interventions could inform future policy and program development (Alegría et al., 2018).

Methodological challenges and inconsistent findings prevent a definitive understanding of which social determinants should be addressed to improve mental health outcomes and within what populations these interventions may be most effective. Future research must include longitudinal, population-based designs to identify risk factors associated with the disorder that contribute to its causation (Brander et al., 2016). Recent advances in strategies to collect and analyze data on social determinants suggest the potential to better appraise their impact and to implement interventions (Alegría et al., 2018). There is also a need for longitudinal studies assessing quality of life of both children and families over the life course of childhood-onset conditions like OCD, and studies of both clinical and community samples with sufficient power to examine sociodemographic and clinical variables together.

Conclusions

The gap between the number of people with mental disorders and the number treated represents a major Canadian and global public health challenge (Evans-Lacko et al., 2018). Individual-level early childhood interventions, as well as policies addressing socio-economic inequalities at a societal level, are needed to improve mental health in childhood and adolescence. The impacts of familial and environmental factors affecting the symptoms, diagnosis, and outcomes of mental disorders among children and youth from diverse geographic regions and cultural groups within Canada have not been well characterized, particularly for disorders such as OCD. An increased understanding of these factors – particularly in the context of common environmental and socio-economic threats such as the COVID-19 pandemic – represent important opportunities for further research.

Increasing evidence suggests that social determinants of health may influence the recognition of symptoms of mental disorders, symptom severity, symptom content, help-seeking, barriers to care, the evidence base for informing treatment, and quality of life. Early treatment of conditions, such as OCD, has the potential to effectively alter a child's developmental trajectory with outcomes that are apparently more optimistic than for adults. However, delays in treatment are common and multiple barriers to access represent a significant public health priority.

Populations made vulnerable by poverty, social inequity, and discrimination undoubtedly experience poorer long-term mental and physical health outcomes, but more work is required to understand the social factors affecting management of mental health disorders in Canadian children, and factors contributing to resiliency. Coordinated efforts by clinicians, practitioners, service providers, researchers, and policymakers to reduce the burden of mental illnesses, like OCD, must consider risk and protective factors that act at the level of the individual, family, community, and population. Interventions aimed at educating the public and health care providers, destigmatizing mental illness, improving family function and distress, and establishing more accessible and economic treatment formats are critical priorities in decreasing the national burden of childhood-onset psychiatric disorders.

4 Mental Health Risks among Immigrant and Refugee Children in Canada

BUKOLA SALAMI, DOMINIC A. ALAAZI,
AND CARLA HILARIO

Migration is a growing global phenomenon. The International Organization for Migration (IOM) estimates 244 million international migrants worldwide, many of whom have settled in urban areas of high-income countries (IOM, 2018). Approximately 31 million of these migrants are children (UNICEF, 2018). While the majority of child migrants are not refugees, around 41 to 51 per cent of refugees are children (IOM, 2018). An estimated one-third of children living outside their country of birth are refugees, often with pre-migration experiences that pose challenges to their mental health. In 2016, over 7.5 million people in Canada – or 21.9 per cent of the population – were immigrants, including children (Statistics Canada, 2017a). In 2016, 2.2 million children in Canada were either foreign-born or had parents who were foreign-born. This demographic represented 37.5 per cent of Canadian children in 2016, up from 34.6 per cent in 2011. Children migrate to Canada for diverse reasons, including family reunion and displacement by war and violence.

Mental health is a growing concern among immigrant children and youth in Canada. Pre-migration factors (e.g., experiences of war and violence) and post-migration factors (e.g., racism, discrimination, and barriers to health care) can contribute to poor mental health outcomes for immigrant children. In this chapter, we draw upon our own research and the Canadian and international literature to examine mental health determinants among immigrants in general, and among African immigrant[1] children in particular.

---

1 In this chapter, the term "African immigrants" is interchangeably invoked with the term "Black Canadians." While there are similarities between the two terms, it is recognized that there are differences between these two groups. Not all African immigrants are Black, and not all Black Canadians are African immigrants. Terms were employed as utilized in cited studies. Terms were also selected based on inclusion and exclusion criteria for the relevant research project discussed in this chapter.

Mental Health of Immigrants in Canada

Cumulative evidence suggests that immigrants arrive in Canada healthier than the average Canadian (Lu & Ng, 2019; Vang et al., 2017). However, their health deteriorates after some time in Canada. This phenomenon, termed the "healthy immigrant effect," is well-documented in the literature, and thus requires no further elaboration. It is crucial, however, to mention that its dimensions extend beyond physical health indicators to encompass mental wellness as well. Studies worldwide point to increased risk of mental health problems and illnesses in immigrant groups (Belhadj Kouider et al., 2015; Bourque et al., 2011; Foo et al., 2018).

In Canada, mental health problems and illnesses are more prevalent in some immigrant groups than others, with refugee populations being the most affected. The Canadian Community Health Survey (CCHS) points to lower rates of psychiatric disorders (e.g., depression and bipolar disorder) among first-generation economic immigrants (Akhtar-Danesh & Landeen, 2007; Ali, 2002; Menezes et al., 2011; Schaffer et al., 2009; Stafford et al., 2011). However, Canadian studies do not concur with this position. For instance, a study of Ethiopian immigrant youth in Toronto reported a 9.8 per cent lifetime prevalence rate of depression (Fenta et al., 2004), which was slightly higher than the national average of between 7.9 and 8.6 per cent (Mood Disorders Society of Canada, 2007). Higher rates of mental health disorders within immigrant populations have also been reported in studies conducted in Nova Scotia and Quebec (Kisely et al., 2008; Mechakra-Tahiri et al., 2007; Tousignant et al., 1999). However, only a limited number of Canadian-wide studies have been conducted (McDermott et al., 2007). In contrast to economic immigrants, refugees experience poorer mental health outcomes, particularly in the initial years following migration.

Mental Health of Immigrant Populations in Canada

Our research team used the Canadian Mental Health Survey to analyze the mental health of immigrants and non-immigrants in Canada (Salami, Yakskina et el., 2017). This national study indicated no statistically significant differences in self-perceived mental health or in the diagnosis of mood disorders of immigrants and non-immigrants aged fifteen to seventy-nine years. However, immigrants' mental health was strongly associated with time since migration, age, and socio-economic status. Immigrants who had lived in Canada for less than five years had better mental health status than immigrants who had lived in Canada for ten years or more. For instance, recent immigrants (less than five years in Canada) were nearly four times more likely to report better mental health. This effect attenuated with longer duration of stay in Canada. Our analysis further indicated that immigrant youth had poorer mental health status than adult immigrants. These findings have been corroborated by qualitative research findings. Interviews with fifty-three immigrant service providers in Alberta revealed an elevated risk of mental health problems for immigrant children and youth, who additionally face some of the most formidable barriers to mental health services and supports (Salami, Hegadoren et al., 2017). Some of these risks include cultural conflicts and family dynamics across transnational spaces. Family dynamics and parenting practices have been demonstrated as playing a crucial role in child mental health by, for example, moderating access to emotional and material supports. Similarly, cultural conflicts experienced by immigrant adolescents during the formation of their identities also pose a risk to youth mental health.

The findings from our analysis of the Canadian Health Measures Survey are consistent with previous studies that point to poorer mental health status for younger immigrants than for older ones (Fenta et al., 2004; Pahwa et al., 2012). Similarly, the Mental Health Commission of Canada (MHCC) notes that mental health problems are more common among younger populations than older populations (MHCC, 2013). Based on their analysis of the National Population Health Survey, Pahwa et al. (2012) noted a need for ethnically targeted research, policies, and programs that focus on immigrant children.

Age at migration has been associated with risk of mental health disorders (Islam, 2015; Patterson et al., 2013). Immigrants who arrived in Canada prior to age 6 reported the highest risk for mood, anxiety, and substance use disorders (Islam, 2015; Patterson et al., 2013). A study by Kwak and Rudmin (2014) found that younger adolescents (12 to 14 years) reported poorer mental health status than older adolescents (18 to 19 years). In relation to boys, the age gradient in risk of mental disorders was more intense in younger girls, who reported greater stress and chronic psychosomatic illnesses than older girls. However, despite these observations, immigrant adolescents were found to have better mental health status than non-immigrant adolescents (Kwak & Rudmin, 2014). Further studies by Kwak (2016) found that second- and third-generation immigrant children have poorer mental health status than their first-generation counterparts. Differences in mental health status among immigrant groups are also influenced by gender and ethnicity. According to a recent report on immigrant children in Canada from Hong Kong, China, and the Philippines, levels of emotional distress among immigrant children vary considerably, with Hong Kongese children being the most severely affected, and Filipino children being the least affected; children of Chinese background were only moderately affected (Beiser et al., 2014). A systematic review of emotional and behavioural problems in migrant children and adolescents in North America found that Asian immigrant children had higher rates of emotional and behavioural problems than other immigrant children (Belhadj Kouider et al., 2015). Other studies also identified a higher prevalence of mental health problems in some immigrant children than in non-immigrant children. Tousignant et al. (1999), for example, found that refugees aged 12 to 19 years had an elevated prevalence of major depression and dysthymia compared to other Quebecois adolescents. Thus, reported rates of mental health problems in immigrant children in Canada vary according to age, ethnicity, and pre-migration experiences (Guruge & Butt, 2015; Hansson et al., 2012).

Social Determinants of Mental Health among African Immigrant Children in Canada

African immigrant children and youth experience some of the worst social and mental health outcomes in Canada (Kon et al., 2012; Maimann, 2014; Saunders, Gill et al., 2018). In a recent Canadian study, African-Canadians (including immigrants) constituted the highest proportion of youth presenting with mental health crises at emergency rooms (Saunders, Gill et al., 2018). At 25 per cent, African-Canadians were also disproportionately represented in youth gangs across Canada (Public Safety Canada, 2007). Research evidence points to pre-emigration, sociocultural, and structural determinants of the mental health of African immigrant children in Canada. Ranging from cultural practices of child discipline to poverty and racism, these determinants demonstrate intricacies and an interconnectedness that present complex challenges to mental health practitioners and policy makers.

PRE-EMIGRATION TRAUMAS

Over the past several decades, many African immigrants arriving in Canada have come from refugee backgrounds, with potentially elevated levels of war-related trauma, depression, and psychotic disorders (Lincoln et al., 2016). Yet research data on the impact of pre-emigration trauma on African immigrant children and youth in Canada are almost non-existent. However, one recent qualitative study found that despite several years of stay in Canada, African immigrant youth from war-affected countries have continued to experience "flashbacks" of the horrors of armed conflicts (Woodgate & Busolo, 2018). Another Canadian study revealed clinically diagnosed post-traumatic stress disorder among some Sudanese parent participants (Donnelly et al., 2011), which was potentially inimical to their parenting success and to the mental well-being of their children. Our team's ethnographic research revealed frequent reports of trauma-related family dysfunction among African refugees in Alberta (Salami, Okeke-Ihejirika et al., 2017c), as described by two community leaders:

> There are so many things that they need to deal with. Some of them have witnessed violence because of the wars that happened ... that kind of trauma and the violence that they witnessed before they came here. So, those things would contribute to how parents raise their children here. (Community leader 1)
>
> Some people, during the war, they have faced trauma ... I was shot. A bullet entered there and came out here ... A lot of people are actually seeing flashbacks. They are seeing problems. They are traumatized, and it's affecting ... relationships at home. It's affecting their relationships at work. Sometimes they can be angry, because some of these things they've seen. (Community leader 2)

Trauma-related family dysfunctionality adversely affects the quality of parent-child relationships and the ability of parents to create social and material conditions that support child mental development. Accordingly, mental health interventions for war-affected immigrant children must also address the pre-emigration mental health experiences of their parents. Indeed, the international literature is awash with claims of a causal relationship between parents' post-traumatic stress disorder and their children's psychological stress (Herring et al., 2006; Lambert et al., 2014; Ostrowski et al., 2007). This understanding, along with our ethnographic data, leads us to suggest that pre-migration trauma is an important determinant of African immigrant child mental health, especially when past trauma is continually reinforced through parents' post-traumatic stress disorder and family dysfunctionality (Salami, Okeke-Ihejirika et al., 2017). Yet, the Canadian health care system's response to this growing mental health epidemic has been slow, in part due to the insufficiency of pertinent mental health data and resources across Canada.

STRUCTURAL DETERMINANTS

Several structural factors converge to produce post-migration psychosocial stress for African immigrant families. Across Canada, African immigrants encounter oppressive systems of institutional relations and practices that elevate their experiences of psychosocial stress. For example, racism and racial discrimination against African immigrants are commonplace in the Canadian labour market (Creese & Wiebe, 2012; Danso, 2002). Consequently, the majority of African immigrants work longer hours in low-skilled and minimum wage jobs, despite possessing educational and professional credentials that are comparable to and in some instances better than the qualifications of their Canadian-born counterparts (Creese & Wiebe, 2012; Opoku-Dapaah, 2006). Using data from the 2006 Census, Fearon and Wald (2011) found that Black Canadian workers had incomes 13.7 per cent lower than the incomes earned by White Canadian workers. "Wage discrimination and occupational segregation" (p. 324) remained a strong predictor of the earning gap after controlling for other wage-determining factors in their statistical model. Data from the 2016 Census also show that, in 2015, first-generation Black immigrants earned sixty-eight cents for every one dollar non-racialized workers earned (Block et al., 2019), which represents a much wider earnings gap over the 2006 figure. This form of discrimination creates economic hardships, material deprivation, and psychological stress for African immigrant families in ways that affect parent-child relations and ultimately child mental health outcomes (Simich et al., 2010). Employment discrimination can further exacerbate existing patterns of socio-economic inequalities between African immigrants and their Canadian counterparts. Our ethnographic research (Salami, Okeke-Ihejirika et al., 2017) with African immigrant parents and community leaders in Alberta indicated that African immigrant youth who lived in poverty-affected and financially distressed households had a greater tendency to drop out of school and to experience drug and gang-related violence.

Economic hardships and material deprivation are not the only proximate determinants of poor mental health outcomes among African immigrant children. Canadian institutional practices, especially in the school system, have also been implicated in the social production of mental health problems for African immigrant children and youth. Through unfair and culturally inconsiderate school practices, such as standardized English language proficiency tests, many African immigrant children have been dismissively portrayed as having communication disorders and learning disabilities (Usman, 2012), causing them unbearable embarrassment and emotional distress. Our research in Alberta encountered reports of teachers attempting to nudge African immigrant children towards vocational and other less desirable career options that require less rigorous academic training (Salami, Okeke-Ihejirika et al., 2017).

Moreover, racism against African and other immigrant families is rife in the Canadian housing market. Immigrants experience struggles finding appropriate housing (Francis, 2010; Mensah & Williams, 2013; Teixeira,

2008). The risk of housing instability and homelessness is reportedly high among African immigrants, particularly those from refugee backgrounds (Francis, 2009). These discriminatory practices have contributed to the segregation of African immigrant families, most of whom reside in economically deprived and crime-ridden inner-city neighbourhoods across Canada (Anisef et al., 2010; Carter et al., 2009). Children are some of the most conspicuous victims of housing stress in North America. Research conducted in the US demonstrates a positive correlation between housing stress and behavioural problems in children (Evans et al., 2001; Singh & Ghandour, 2012). Data on the health effects of housing stress in African immigrant children in Canada are scant. However, anecdotal evidence in Canada suggests precarious housing and unemployment as primers for psychosocial stress in African immigrant parents and children. For example, Danso (2002) documented how housing precariousness and unemployment have driven African immigrants in Toronto into despair and towards suicidal behaviours. As research on the health effects of housing stress in African immigrant children in Canada is inconclusive, there is an imperative to improve our understanding of the impacts of housing insecurity on this demographic.

Racism in child welfare practices presents another major challenge to mental health among African immigrant children. Across Canada, teachers, social workers, and medical practitioners demonstrate a higher tendency to refer African immigrant children to child protective services. These referrals often result in the removal of African immigrant children from their homes and their admission into foster care. Today, African and Black immigrant children are over-represented in Canada's child welfare system. For example, African and Black immigrant children constitute 41 per cent of children and youth in Toronto's child protective system, although this demographic represents only 8 per cent of the city's total population (CityNews, 2016). The removal from and subsequent loss of bond with biological family has adverse mental health implications for fostered children. For example, compared to other children, African immigrant children ageing out of foster care have a higher risk of school dropout, homelessness, teenage pregnancy, and encounters with the criminal justice system (Ontario Association of Children's Aid Societies, 2015).

SOCIOCULTURAL DETERMINANTS

For a significant number of African immigrant families, the resettlement process entails learning and adjusting to new norms of social behaviour, a step in the integration trajectory that comes more naturally to children than to parents. Children are usually the first to learn English, to make friends, and to adopt Western values and lifestyles. These changes are often a major source of parent-child conflicts in African immigrant families, especially when such changes create concerns about cultural assimilation and loss of cultural identity. Cultural conflicts between immigrant parents and their children are a precursor for child mental health problems. Among African immigrant families in Canada, such conflicts contribute to emotional and internalizing problems in African immigrant children and youth (Beiser et al., 2012). Most of these conflicts arise from the disciplinary practices of parents and their need to cultivate strong cultural values in their children (Alaazi et al., 2018; Hassan & Rousseau, 2009; Makwarimba et al., 2013). A parent in one of our studies (Salami, Okeke-Ihejirika et al., 2017) reveals an example of this sort of cultural tension in African immigrant families:

> I know the story for a boy ... He was so difficult. He came from Africa, and he was really, really difficult to manage ... It was conflict every time between the mother and the boy. And they finally returned the boy to Ivory Coast, because they couldn't [manage him] ... he called 911 and the father was really, really concerned about losing his job and all. So, he decided to send him back to Africa until he gets really good. (Parent)

Although transnational foster-parenting is a popular parental response to cultural conflicts between parents and children, this practice can have serious mental health implications for children, including experiences of depression (Suârez-Orozco et al., 2002). For families that remain intact in the face of family conflicts, the incursion of two diametrically opposed cultures (Western versus African) can inadvertently produce psychosocial confliction for African immigrant children as they struggle to gain social acceptance within their foster families and the wider society in which they now live and conduct their daily lives. This maneuvering often involves attempts at blending Western and African value systems and norms of behaviour. Several African community leaders in one of our studies identified psychosocial confliction as being detrimental to the mental health of African immigrant children (Salami, Okeke-Ihejirika et al., 2017).

Although family supports, social relationships, and education advancement play a protective role against adverse child mental health outcomes (Hall-Lande et al., 2007; Wille et al., 2008), there is evidence suggesting that most African immigrant children in Canada lack such protective mechanisms. Moreover, many African immigrant children experience isolation from school peers due to their skin colour (Woodgate & Busolo, 2018). Codjoe (2001) documented the struggles of a sample of African immigrant high school students in Alberta and noted a high prevalence of racist name-calling, peer bullying, and school practices that alienate and undermine their academic success. Not only do African immigrant children and youth across Canada leave school due to negative school practices (Anisef et al., 2010), but they also experience social isolation, loneliness, and emotional problems, which place them at a greater risk of suicide (Calati et al., 2018; Codjoe, 2001; Hall-Lande et al., 2007).

SERVICE UTILIZATION

Despite reports of mental health challenges among African immigrant families in Canada (Fenta et al., 2004), the utilization of mental health services by these families is comparatively low (Fenta et al., 2006, 2007). Recent data from Ontario suggest comparatively lower per capita consumption costs of mental health services for immigrants and refugees from sub-Saharan Africa than for the non-immigrant population (McKenzie et al., 2016). Both cultural and structural factors account for the limited contact of African immigrants with professional mental health care. Culturally, African immigrants may deny and even stigmatize experiences of mental health problems. Our research with African immigrant families in Alberta (Salami et al., 2017c) revealed a tendency to frame mental health as a taboo topic which is almost never discussed, and showed that remedies to mental health problems are not always proffered:

> In my community, mental health is kind of taboo ... they don't talk about it that much. Even if the child has [mental health problems], maybe you can sense it and you can tell from the behaviour or something, but the majority of the parents won't tell you. (Parent)
> ... in my community, two youth killed themselves. And if you ask me, did we say it aloud? No, we didn't ... we haven't said it out loud ... because it is a taboo to talk about mental state, that we're not doing well mentally. (Settlement service worker)

In rare instances where there is acknowledgement of mental health problems, treatment emphasis tends to focus more on spiritual rather than professional care (Fenta et al., 2006). Cultural adaptation of mental health services has not yet occurred in Canada. As such, cultural barriers to mental health services and supports exist for African immigrant families. African community leaders and African immigrant parents in one of our studies (Salami, Okeke-Ihejirika et al., 2017) expressed dissatisfaction with perceived cultural insensitivity across a range of social services in Alberta. The cultural gap in service provision in Canada persists, despite suggestions for incorporation of immigrants' beliefs, values, and practices in service provision (M. Stewart, Kushner et al., 2017).

In summary, culture, race, and social class interact to produce complex mental health challenges for African immigrant children and youth in Canada. The determinants of child mental health among African immigrants demonstrate intricately intertwined political, sociocultural, and structural dimensions. Addressing the mental health challenges of vulnerable African immigrant children requires careful consideration of these multiple determinants and their interactions.

Implications for Research, Practice, and Policy

Existing evidence on the mental health of immigrant and refugee children in Canada suggests the need for ongoing surveillance of and research into patterns of mental health risks in this population. Mental health challenges are more common in younger newcomer populations, with signs and symptoms of some mental illnesses often presenting in youth. Determinants of mental health among immigrant and refugee children require further investigation. Knowledge syntheses from reviews of research on young immigrant groups in Canada can offer valuable insights into determinants of mental health for this population (Hilario, Oliffe et al., 2015). Given the paucity of evidence on pre-migration trauma in refugee children, further research is needed to inform services and programs that ameliorate trauma effects and enhance mental health.

The combination of pre-migration and post-migration social stressors presents unique conditions that may render immigrant and refugee children particularly vulnerable to mental health challenges. Variations in the prevalence of mental illness and emotional distress between immigrant children from different countries suggest a need for tailored programming and service provision responsive to the needs of particular groups. Refugee children, for example, may need specialized services given the higher likelihood of their exposure to pre-migration stressors and trauma from witnessing political violence or as a result of displacement. Effective screening and assessment of pre-migration traumas is needed to determine mental health risk, especially among refugee children.

Structural determinants of mental health among African immigrant families present practice and policy-level opportunities focused on anti-racism in the labour and housing markets. Research suggests that African immigrants face racial discrimination that contributes to underemployment, poorer working conditions, and lower wages, which in turn leads to economic hardships and stress for African immigrant families. There is emerging evidence to suggest the existence of relationships between these factors and the social and health outcomes of African immigrant children and youth. African immigrant families are forced to find housing in poorer neighbourhoods due to unemployment and low incomes – a combination that contributes to psychosocial stress for immigrants and their children. Given documented linkages between housing stress and mental health, government policies that promote housing affordability can have downstream positive impacts on the mental health of African immigrant children.

Compared to children of other racial backgrounds, African and Black immigrant children have a higher risk of being removed from their families. African immigrant parents are investigated twice as often as other families for child abuse. The evidence from across Canada demonstrates a clear racial gradient in family contact with child protective services, with African, Black, and Indigenous families being the most unfairly treated. There is thus a need to deracialize child protective practices and to address the over-representation of African immigrant children in foster care. Allocating public funding to create safe spaces and community parenting supports for African immigrant families can further help to address the disproportionate presence of African immigrant children in foster care across the country.

Current evidence also reveals relationships between mental health programs and factors such as gender and ethnicity. Recent evidence suggests that immigrant girls face a higher mental health risk compared to immigrant boys. Research using population-based survey data with immigrant youth in Canada demonstrates similar patterns with girls reporting significantly higher rates of extreme levels of stress and despair compared to boys (Hilario et al., 2014). This research suggests a need to consider the role of gender, as well as ethnicity, when designing programs for mental health promotion.

Tailored mental health services and guidelines for health service providers are required to address the unique mental health needs of immigrant children (Hilario, Vo et al., 2015). Policies are also needed to assure funding and to provide guidance for the development, implementation, and evaluation of relevant accessible services. A family-centred approach to assessment and treatment may address the impacts of migration and traumas on the entire family, including the potential impacts of parental mental illness on the mental health of their children.

Lastly, there is a need to enhance mental health service utilization among immigrant children and their families to improve early detection and treatment of mental illness. This requires programs that diminish the stigma attached to mental illness in some countries of origin, and the development of culturally tailored and responsive services that consider newcomers' beliefs, values, and practices. Addressing the mental health challenges faced by immigrant and refugee children in Canada requires multi-pronged interventions and system changes that account for multiple, intersecting determinants of their mental health.

SECTION II

Adolescents' Experiences

Section II Introduction: Adolescents' Experiences

JOCELYN EDEY

Many of Canada's youth face complex social conditions that increase their risk for health problems. Adolescents' development and growth stages and circumstances are significantly different from children and adults, and require a concentrated focus to effectively address their unique risks, strengths, and needs. Addressing knowledge gaps regarding social determinants and risk and protective factors affecting adolescents could inform the creation of supportive interventions and programs.

This section begins with a discussion of adolescents living in low-income circumstances and facing additional challenges of coping with respiratory health conditions. Chapter 5, "Low-Income Adolescents Living with Respiratory Challenges," provides insights into socio-economic influences on adolescent health and interventions to alleviate such influences. The perspectives of adolescents living in poverty are shared, including the challenges of coping with peer pressure and facing the dual stigma of poverty and chronic illness. Additional concerns facing these youth include feelings of isolation and desire for social inclusion. An intervention for low-income youth was designed that focused on bridging support gaps in low-income youths' changing repertoire. The impacts of this intervention will be presented, along with recommendations for future programs for vulnerable youth.

Chapter 6, "Fostering Support for Indigenous Adolescents Facing Health Inequities," introduces the complexities of factors influencing the health of Indigenous peoples and the fact that Indigenous peoples in Canada experience poorer health outcomes and inequitable access to health services relative to non-Indigenous populations. Chapter 6 will explore the experiences of Indigenous adolescents with respiratory conditions and salient support strategies. This chapter will emphasize the importance of culturally appropriate care, Indigenous health indicators to monitor programs, and health equity for Indigenous youth.

Indigenous approaches to knowledge, including Two-eyed Seeing, Ethical Space, and Indigenous ways of knowing, that influence current and future research and services will also be introduced. Promising health programs focused on diabetes reduction (e.g., Indigenous Youth Mentorship program) and sexual health promotion (e.g., CheckUp project) for Indigenous adolescents are highlighted. Recommendations for connectivity to culture, language, and land; restoration of positive Indigeneity; and self-determination are provided.

Chapter 7, "Supporting Refugee Adolescents," is the final chapter in this section and will focus on a different vulnerable group: Syrian refugee adolescents. Chapter 4 introduced the mental health problems of refugees that rise as Canada continues to welcome high numbers of newcomers who face risk factors that make them vulnerable to mental and physical health problems. Canadian documents confirm major mental health risks for refugee adolescents and deficits in cultural appropriateness and accessibility of services and supports. Chapter 7 will share insights from a recent nationally funded study that tested social and cultural impacts of an accessible technology-based support intervention for Syrian refugee adolescents in Canada. A support intervention will be presented that aims to decrease loneliness and isolation, and increase self-confidence, knowledge of opportunities and resources, and coping strategies.

This section focuses on factors such as ethnicity, socio-economic status, and migration status, each of which can contribute to the development of health problems for adolescents and influence the prioritization of targeted interventions (World Health Organization, 2014). Examining the risk factors, challenges, and strengths of adolescents can inform program planners and policymakers in identification of strategies that reduce opportunity inequalities and improve adolescent health (Cappa & Giulivi, 2019).

5 Low-Income Adolescents Living with Respiratory Challenges

MIRIAM J. STEWART

Over 4.5 million people (13 per cent) in Canada are considered to be low-income and almost a million of these people are under eighteen years old (Statistics Canada, 2017b). The low-income rate was substantially higher for children with two or more siblings than for a single child in a two-parent family. Among children who lived in a lone-parent family with one child, the low-income rate was 30.5 per cent. This rate increased to 37.2 per cent when there were two children in a single-parent family, and to 55.1 per cent with three or more children (Statistics Canada, 2017b).

Youth aged ten to nineteen who lived in the lowest-income neighbourhoods were twice as likely to have lung problems than youth in higher-income neighbourhoods (Canadian Institute for Health Information, 2018). Low-income youth with asthma were susceptible to more hospitalizations, lower use of other health services (To et al., 2009), and higher rates of non-adherence to a medication regimen (Blais et al., 2006) than higher-income youth. Increased incidence of respiratory health problems among low-income adolescents can exert significant negative impacts on affected youth and their parents, including physical and psychosocial health problems, diminished quality of life, and social isolation. This area of inquiry deserves attention as the burdens of poverty are often compounded by health problems like respiratory illness, and, reciprocally, respiratory problems augment the economic and social burdens facing adolescents, which affect their journey towards adulthood.

There has been insufficient capacity in health systems and communities to diminish respiratory health inequities through targeted supports. A review conducted by our research team revealed major gaps in research focused on respiratory problems experienced by low-income teens. The diverse challenges and barriers experienced by youth coping with both poverty and respiratory problems had not been studied prior to the projects presented in this chapter. The aim of this chapter is to share insights regarding provision of support, guidance, and information to reduce inequity of this high-risk population.

This chapter shares insights from two studies created to support low-income youth living with respiratory health challenges in Canada. One study assessed the needs and preferences of adolescents regarding support programs and services. The second study was designed to pilot test an accessible intervention that provided support and education to low-income adolescents affected by asthma, using an innovative online delivery modality. The perspectives of youth participants are shared in this chapter, in addition to the reported impacts of this pilot intervention.

Support Needs and Preferences of Low-Income Youth

The initial study (M. Stewart, Evans et al., 2016) investigated available programs and services for low-income youth, and their preferences for supportive interventions. Purposive sampling was used to identify potential participants representing varied low-income situations (e.g., working poor, social assistance recipients, unemployed, homeless) and key demographic characteristics such as gender, ethnicity, immigration status, and age that may influence low-income status. Adolescents from two large urban cities in Western Canada participated. At the time of this study, 88,000 people in Winnipeg, Manitoba, and 109,000 people in Edmonton, Alberta lived in poverty (Statistics Canada, 2013c).

Participants were recruited through community service agencies, community networks, child health clinics, voluntary organizations, and food banks serving low-income people. The most effective recruitment tool was flyer delivery to low-income housing complexes. The Statistics Canada Low-Income Cut-Offs (Statistics Canada, 2013d) were used to determine income status of adolescents. Eligibility criteria for inclusion as study participants, in addition to low-income, were older children/ young adolescents (in Grades 5–10 to ensure sufficient developmental maturity for interviews) with physician diagnosis of severe asthma, cystic fibrosis, or other chronic respiratory health conditions (M. Stewart Letourneau et al., 2012).

Thirty-two youth who lived in low-income homes (twenty-one in Edmonton, eleven in Winnipeg) were interviewed. More than 70 per cent of all participants lived in subsidized or low-income housing. The average age was 12.2 years (male: 11.4 years, female: 13.4 years). There were seventeen males (53 per cent) and fifteen females (47 per cent). Almost half of the participants (49 per cent) represented ethnic minorities that included Indigenous (First Nation, Métis), African, African-American, and Asian (Filipino, Chinese). Group interviews were conducted to discuss available programs and services and the types of support programs desired by these youth.

Adolescents described the context of their lives, current challenges, and past experiences. Exemplar quotations from our studies will be presented to highlight the perspectives of youth living with poverty and lung problems. Although some adolescent participants understood causes, symptoms, treatments, and preventive actions, many were not aware of important information that could help them cope effectively with chronic respiratory conditions. Without support and education from health professionals, many low-income youths did not understand the causes and management of their health challenges. To illustrate, many adolescents believed that asthma is episodic and that medication is required only when symptoms appear. One youth described an ambivalent experience with health education:

> I remember I had an allergic reaction and was in the hospital and that nurse showed me how to use [my puffer] ... I have the booklet they gave me still. What I like the best is that it tells me what to do if I'm having an allergic reaction and who I can talk to and [what I like] the least, sometimes it doesn't say what's actually happening to me.

Some teens did not disclose their health condition to others and did not want special treatment. Adolescents wanted to participate in sports, attend school regularly, and have friends, but their respiratory conditions posed barriers. Most youth thought that missing school and exclusion from physical education, sports, or games because of breathing difficulties made them different from their peers. These adolescents believed that the combination of low-income and asthma or allergies made them less like their peers: "I don't feel like my friends are judging me, I'm just worried that they are." Youth reported that they were more willing to tolerate discomfort due to exacerbation of symptoms, rather than ask friends to stop smoking or request "special treatment." One pre-teen acknowledged that although smoking could have a detrimental effect on his lung condition, it was a strategy to fit in with his peers. Two low-income youth with asthma discussed being different:

> FIRST YOUTH: Having cold-induced asthma, when you are bundled up like the Michelin man, when ... everyone else is wearing miniskirts and flip flops in the middle of winter ... it's just hard to be understood ... And

> every time you walk into school wearing snow pants they're like "no one wears snow pants anymore" and then everyone looks at you like you, like you're ...
>
> SECOND YOUTH: ... weird or something.

Several adolescents avoided alarming family and friends who "freaked out" when they had trouble breathing. Some youth were excluded or even harassed by their peers. Teens wanted peers to understand why they could not compete in sports or participate in other physical activities. These adolescents also wished other people would respond appropriately when their lung problems were exacerbated, as clarified in this conversation between two low-income adolescents:

> FIRST ADOLESCENT: It sucks being labelled for your illness and then being labelled for being the slowest person, and just because having an illness, or like, not being able to accomplish what other people can do ... they'll say like, "you're slow" or "you suck at doing this" or ... 'cause I can't run as fast as they can without having a coughing fit or I can't, even in track and field too, like I can't do the stuff that other people can, and then I have to sit out for some of the stuff. And then people just call me names and stuff, and then it's unfair because it's not really your choice to have asthma, you're ...
>
> SECOND ADOLESCENT: ... born that way.

Adolescents did not tell peers about their health challenges to avoid feeling different and drawing attention to those differences. Although they desired inclusion, they were often excluded from sports, games, or activities because of breathing problems. Youth wanted peers to understand the barriers that respiratory problems pose to participation, as well as their symptoms and suitable treatment.

Some low-income teens coped with dual burdens of feeling responsible for their family's financial troubles, in addition to having a respiratory condition. Numerous adolescents expressed concern about the negative effects of poor air quality in low-income housing on their health. Many youths indicated that they used rescue inhalers, nebulizers, or steroids only in emergency situations rather than more expensive controller medications. Some inner-city youth indicated that when their inhalers emptied, they would see a physician who would give them free refills.

Participants explained that they wanted support from school classmates and teachers, friends, and their community. Older youth, based on their experience as younger teens, reported that they would prefer a support program that helped them develop confidence and skills needed to independently ask questions about allergen risks (M. Stewart, Letourneau et al., 2012). Support from adolescent peers who were knowledgeable about their health problem was desired. Youth expressed interest in connecting with other low-income teens living with chronic respiratory conditions. Participants explained that a supportive intervention should combine enjoyable, fun activities with learning about their health conditions: "It would make my life better ... Feel like a better person and not feeling so down about yourself 'cause you have no friends and you're asthmatic."

Low-income adolescents often preferred to hide their condition. Misunderstandings about respiratory conditions and associated impacts on physical activities led to feelings of isolation. These low-income youths' perceptions of peer pressure resulted in risk-taking behaviors to hide their illness, such as non-adherence to health regimens. Low-income teens preferred support from peers with experiential knowledge of both their health conditions and poverty. Support from experienced peers, in combination with health professional guidance and knowledge about pulmonary health, could help reduce inequities for this high-risk population.

Support Interventions for Low-Income Youth

This study was designed to pilot test interventions that provide support and education, using computers and telephones, for low-income youth who have asthma. Thirty-three participants were drawn from low-income populations throughout Canada, including Ontario, Alberta, British Columbia, and Nova Scotia. Low-income was determined using Statistics Canada (2015) low-income cut-offs. Their ethnicity encompassed Indigenous (including Métis), African (Zimbabwean, Ugandan, Liberian, Sudanese), African-American, Caucasian, and Asian (Filipino, Chinese). The majority of children/adolescents indicated they had asthma (90.9 per cent). The average attendance in this support intervention for these low-income adolescents was 83.25 per cent.

An eight-session (weekly or biweekly) support–education intervention was conducted over a three-month period. The intervention was implemented online using a secure platform (GoToMeeting©). The sessions were co-facilitated by low-income peer mentors and health professionals who had received prior training. As many low-income families did not have computers or internet access, Chromebooks were provided along with internet sticks.

Qualitative data on the intervention program and process were collected through online session recordings and field notes, written weekly by health professional mentors and peer mentors. Group interviews and individual interviews ($n = 23$) with adolescents conducted at post-test, yielded qualitative data on perceived impacts of the intervention, factors influencing its impacts, satisfaction with the intervention, and recommended changes. In addition, in-depth interviews proceeded with peer mentors and health professionals. Quantitative data on health-related outcomes were elicited using six standardized measures administered pre-intervention and post-intervention to these adolescent participants via telephone.

The reported effects of this support-education intervention for low-income youth affected by respiratory conditions included decreased loneliness and isolation; increased support–seeking coping; expanded social networks; enhanced quality of life and self-confidence; and more appropriate use of health services. Teens' knowledge regarding management of asthma and allergies increased. Youth participants' coping improved despite low-income circumstances.

The use of innovative technology made it possible to offer meetings over a wide geographical area and to manage challenges of different time zones across Canada. Youth participants reported that the online support sessions were interesting and important. They learned from the personal experiences of peer mentors and information provided by health professionals. One teen explained:

> Well, the first session I felt really nervous, and I didn't think that like more than five people, including myself, would be in the sessions, and then I noticed that lots of people weren't afraid [to] step up, and say, I have asthma or allergies or both, and I want to talk about [this] with other kids and adults and see ... how I can like kind of stop myself from having the attacks more than I really need to.

Another low-income youth described how a peer mentor was helpful to him:

> In many ways my chats with [peer mentor] ... were helpful because ... I found out a lot of different information that I might not have known before (like to check my expiry date on my inhalers) ... it just really helped me with knowing that it's okay to have asthma and allergies, and you don't need to feel ashamed of it cause like [peer mentor] has it, like everyone in the asthma and allergy course either has asthma or allergies or both. I found [support program] really helpful.

Getting to know other low-income adolescents who shared the same challenges, problems, and issues was a critical component of the success of this pilot support intervention. Building relationships and sharing knowledge with peers helped youth feel less lonely. Most teens mentioned that they had previously felt alone because they did not know anyone their age suffering from asthma and allergies. As two teen participants explained: "I feel good today because I'm not the only one that has asthma," and "I know that there are many more people in the world than I thought that had asthma or allergies or both and ... I don't feel like I'm alone ... because many other people in the world have these asthma and allergy problems."

Diminished loneliness was also suggested in a paired-samples t-test of the Loneliness and Social Dissatisfaction Questionnaire for Young Children (Cassidy & Asher, 1992). The post-intervention test score on loneliness was slightly lower ($M = 19.9$, $SD = 3.62$) than the pre-intervention test score ($M = 20.15$, $SD = 2.06$; $t\,12 = 0.25$, $p = 0.40$), although the decrease was statistically non-significant.

Youth participants appreciated information received from this support-education program. Many adolescents did not have adequate education about respiratory conditions, including relevant medications, prior to these sessions. These adolescents wanted to know more about causes of their respiratory challenges and ways to prevent symptoms. Teens discussed triggers of asthma and allergies, and strategies used to feel better. Participant feedback about the intervention impacts included:

> Right now I feel happy, because now I know more ways how to avoid getting an asthma attack.
>
> I'm able to talk about my asthma and allergies to people. I feel good knowing that your friends can help you with your problems. I feel happy about my asthma and that I talked about it.
>
> Today's group was good for me because I got to learn about other people, like how other people manage their allergies.
>
> Today's group was good for me because I got to see more triggers for asthma.

Adolescents also were grateful for opportunities to talk with health professionals about their conditions and medications and to share stories about their health challenges.

Many low-income adolescents described lack of support within their school context. Youth participants believed that many teachers were not empathetic when a teen experienced an exacerbation. Youth learned how to educate peers and teachers about their health condition, and how to receive proper care in emergency situations:

> They told me to hold my inhaler straight, and they have also told me like if you're starting to sort of find it a little hard to breathe, and you don't

have your emergency puffers ... if you were at gym at school and you find it hard to breathe cause you were running around, you could just tell your teacher I need to sit out because I'm starting to have an asthma attack.

Perceived support from three sources – family, friends, and significant others – was examined using the Multidimensional Scale of Perceived Social Support (Zimet et al., 1988). Results of a paired-samples t-test indicated that the post-intervention test score for perceived support was slightly higher (M = 75.4, SD = 8.78) than pre-intervention test score (M = 73.33, SD = 6.32; t 11 = −1.08, p = 0.15) although not statistically significant. Low-income teen participants provided emotional support to peers by "being there" and by "just lending an ear" to listen. The youth also supported each other by sharing their life stories, affirming that other teens were dealing with similar situations. Their ideas were valued because peers paid attention to what they were saying during support-group sessions.

Adolescents also shared how having insufficient money and resources impeded their ability to manage their health conditions at home. One youth illustrated how financial constraints posed barriers to buying respiratory medications: "I feel great to have people like you, teach us about allergies and how to contain them, and about money situations, and also that other people are going through what I'm going through." Low-income youth benefited by meeting with other teens dealing with similar issues. This made them feel less isolated. Most participants maintained they had no previous opportunities to meet with peers who had the same health challenges and they had felt socially isolated prior to the support intervention.

The support intervention provided a safe space where adolescents could talk with each other about their experiences. This helped the teens build self-esteem, knowing that they too could overcome similar challenges. In addition, these youth were better equipped to educate other people about their health challenges. The support intervention program created an educational forum in which low-income youth learned about their medical conditions, including causal factors, triggers, and management. Health professionals answered questions and provided medical information. The knowledge gained from these sessions boosted the teens' confidence and self-care ability. Having peer mentors who had personal experience living in poverty and dealing with the same medical conditions motivated them. Support from health professionals and peers reassured them and enhanced their willingness to seek treatment and to manage their health.

Insights and Implications

Accessible respiratory health education resources should be tailored to challenges faced by low-income adolescents from diverse cultural backgrounds (Garwick & Seppelt, 2010). Multilevel, accessible, comprehensive support interventions for youth dealing with poverty (Schofield, 2007) should be flexible (McGhan et al., 2005). Poverty signifies a clustering of disadvantages for several social determinants of children's health (Raphael, 2010). This study illustrates some pathways by which poverty can influence health, including material pathways (e.g., low-income, poor housing conditions), behavioural pathways (e.g., non-adherence, rescue inhalers vs. controller medications), and psychosocial pathways (e.g., limited social participation, stigma). Interventions should be targeted at disrupting the reciprocal cycle of poverty and respiratory illness, while also striving to alleviate the psychosocial impacts of stigma and stressful interactions. This cycle could be interrupted through interventions necessitating collaboration with diverse health-related sectors (M. Stewart, Evans et al., 2016; M. Stewart, King et al., 2013).

Low-income teens with chronic health problems experience loneliness, isolation, and peer pressure that result in risks, such as non-adherence to health regimens (Kyngas, 2004). Adolescents value the support of peers who share similar chronic conditions (Protudjer et al., 2009, 2011). A review of previous studies revealed that interventions typically emphasized education and information, not support; rarely included support from peers; and were hospital/clinic-based using face-to-face modes rather than community-based innovative technology. Research had not addressed the unique support needs and intervention preferences of low-income adolescents with respiratory health problems and had not designed salient supportive interventions for these vulnerable teens. This pilot research demonstrates that online peer support interventions can improve the relevance and uptake of health programs through tailored support strategies, but only if they are informed by participants' preferences and circumstances.

Innovative support interventions for low-income teens have the potential to decrease loneliness and increase perceived social support. Replication and testing of interventions for low-income youth using larger multisite samples are important. Interventions are best targeted at addressing causes of material and social deprivation and social exclusion, while also alleviating the psychosocial impacts of stigma, degradation, and stress related to poverty (M. Stewart, Masuda et al., 2015). Strategies improving access to multilevel community-based support for vulnerable adolescents and their families can inform development of appropriate, effective, and beneficial supports for specific challenges.

6 Fostering Support for Indigenous Adolescents Facing Health Inequities

MALCOLM KING AND ALEXANDRA KING

Introduction

For Canadians in general, living in rural or remote areas decreases opportunities for education, employment, healthy food supply, and access to health care and prevention services. Indigenous peoples in Canada, due to complex legacies of settler colonialism, experience poorer health outcomes and inequitable access to care relative to non-Indigenous populations. Geographic displacement, residential school education, and religious suppression are determinants of disease inequities for Indigenous peoples (Truth and Reconciliation Commission of Canada [TRCC], 2015). The appropriation of traditional land by European settlers and government legislation led to the displacement of many communities from land integral to health and wellness. Compounded by residential schools, the Sixties Scoop (Hanson, 2009), and assimilation forced upon Indigenous children, adolescents, and their families and communities, generations of Indigenous families have suffered from colonial-derived health inequities (TRCC, 2015).

One Indigenous health deficit affecting Indigenous youth is type 2 diabetes, with its early onset and increased levels of severity and complications in young Indigenous people (Crowshoe et al., 2018; Dyck et al., 2010). Mental health issues, as evidenced by addictions and suicides (Harder et al., 2012), are other stark examples of health deficits for Indigenous adolescents, as are sexually transmitted and blood-borne infections (Wexler et al., 2009). Inequities in respiratory health problems among Indigenous adolescents are less well-known, but there is emerging evidence indicating that Indigenous youth are particularly vulnerable to asthma and, importantly, have poorer access to relevant health education and services.

The historical adversity that Indigenous adolescents continue to face calls for resilience-centred interventions that empower youth rather than solely educate them. In the fields of diabetes and mental health, youth empowerment, working with youth, promoting connections with Elders and community, and connecting with land and culture all have positive impacts on these diverse conditions. Thus, it is reasonable to suppose that similar approaches to interventions are relevant to other health conditions.

Foundational Principles

Three foundational principles should be considered in working with Indigenous people of all ages and Indigenous communities in health services and health research: Ethical Space, Two-eyed Seeing, and strengths-based approaches.

Engagement: Ethical Space

Elder and philosopher Willie Ermine (Sturgeon Lake Cree Nation, Saskatchewan) developed the concept of Ethical Space, and its application to research, as part of his master's thesis (Ermine, 2007). Its application is critical to ethical engagement and the development of meaningful and productive relationships between researchers or service providers and the Indigenous communities with which they wish to engage. Ethical Space is an abstract space where two groups of people with different intentions encounter one another (see figure 6.1). It is the space between Western and Indigenous spheres of culture and knowledge relative to health research and services. As individuals, our histories, values, traditions, and world views can significantly affect how we communicate with one another. An ethical, or mutually respectful, zone is a place where different cultures and knowledge systems can engage with one another on equal footing. This provides the opportunity to find solutions to significant health problems that health researchers have not been able to address in conventional ways.

As a conceptual model, there are only two simple spheres representing an Indigenous world view and a Western one. In fact, each sphere is complex because there are many Indigenous world views, as there are many Western world views, and these may come together in a simple one-on-one fashion, or the interactions may be more complex on each side. Important principles embedded in Ethical Space include reciprocity, respect, and humility – recognizing that other ways of knowing have value; that the truths we hold are not the only ones; and that other ways of knowing and seeing the world are legitimate and should be respected.

Figure 6.1. Ethical Space

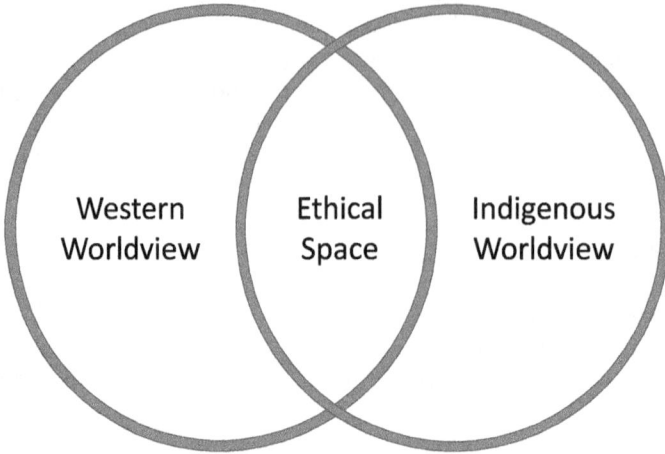

Source: Dr. M. King based on W. Ermine, *The Ethical Space of Engagement* (2007).

Ethical Space has often been referenced back to the famous first treaty that linked European traders and settlers to the Indigenous peoples of eastern North America in the early seventeenth century – the Two-Row Wampum Belt Treaty of 1613, known as *Guswenta* in Mohawk (Venables, 2008). This treaty between the Dutch and the Haudenosaunee (Iroquois) emphasized mutual respect and non-interference between two groups that recognized each other's self-determination. The two rows of purple wampum beads on the belt symbolized the Dutch sailing ship and the Haudenosaunee canoe. The white beads represented peace, friendship, and forever. These symbols translated into this message: "Neither of us will try to steer the other's vessel." In sum, utilizing these principles – respect, equity in relationships, and communities as partners – will ensure a better and more fulfilling engagement in health services and health research.

Two-eyed Seeing

The second principle – Two-eyed Seeing – appears similar to Ethical Space in concept, however, it is more of an operational principle – bringing together and actualizing Indigenous ways of knowing and doing with Western ways of knowing and doing to provide synergy of thought and action towards health. The principle – to see from one eye with the

Figure 6.2. Two-eyed Seeing: *Etuaptmumk* – The perspective of "Two-eyed Seeing," as put forward by Mi'kmaq Elder Albert Marshall

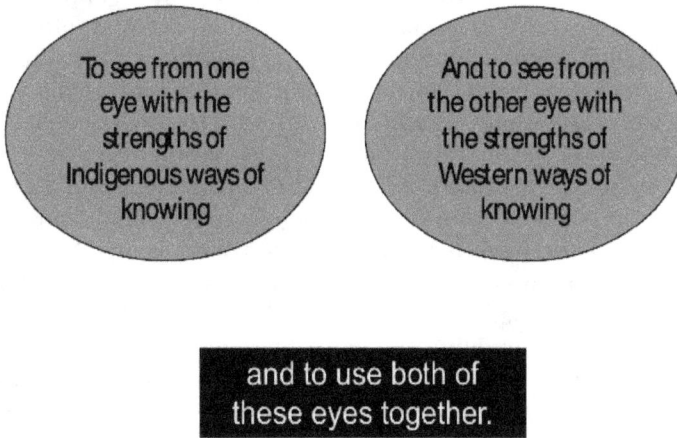

To see from one eye with the strengths of Indigenous ways of knowing

And to see from the other eye with the strengths of Western ways of knowing

and to use both of these eyes together.

Source: Dr. M. King, courtesy of Canadian Institutes of Health Research.

strengths of Indigenous ways of knowing, and to see from the other eye with the strengths of Western ways of knowing, and to use both of these eyes together – involves both seeing (realizing that there are different and potentially complementary strengths in different approaches) and doing (moving from observations to action). The Two-eyed Seeing principle illustrated in figure 3.1 was put forward by Mi'kmaq Elder Albert Marshall (Bartlett et al., 2012), and was adopted by the Canadian Institutes of Health Research (CIHR) as a valid approach to Indigenous health participatory action research (CIHR, 2013). Another representation of Two-eyed Seeing appears in the story of Coyote's Eyes, by American Indian Terry Tafoya (1982), in which Coyote ends up with two very different eyes – that of a mouse and that of a buffalo. Each eye has its strengths, and together they give extraordinary perception.

Strengths-Based Approaches

The third principle is practical – to approach health research and services from a viewpoint of resilience and strength, rather than from a deficit perspective (which sees a problem to be fixed, and which views individuals and communities as passive participants). A strengths-based approach is more active; individuals and their communities are actively involved as participants – from envisioning needs, to formulating approaches, to carrying out the project, to taking a role in interpreting results and disseminating information. Strengths-based approaches are consistent with the participatory principles involved in the Strategy for Patient-Oriented Research developed by the Canadian Institutes of Health Research (CIHR, 2019), and also consistent with the principles of other agencies, such as the International Association for Public Participation. From an Indigenous perspective, principles of collaboration, agency, and empowerment are in line with the self-determination aspects of the United Nations Declaration on the Rights of Indigenous Peoples (United Nations, 2007).

By adopting a strengths-based approach, health goals do not necessarily involve a disease or condition end-point. Most health research and health services are focused on a disease or deficit end-point, whether designing, testing, or implementing interventions, treatments, or preventive measures. However, the main focus of an Indigenous knowledge-development project may be on *wellness* – promoting, maintaining, and re-gaining wellness by itself, or in the context of a variety of health conditions or life circumstances affecting First Nations, Inuit, and Métis peoples. Indigenous health and wellness knowledge/wisdom needs to be awakened or reawakened; however, such knowledge is not yet well-supported given current colonized structures and conceptualizations. Awakening Indigenous health and wellness knowledge will require reconstructing and redeveloping community roles and wellness processes (see figure 6.3). It is within this context that we see the Indigenous community as primary leader, with the academy and the health system as knowledge users.

Where does wellness promotion begin? The physical, mental, emotional, and spiritual end-manifestations can be circumvented by promoting resilient factors at every stage along the path (Fayed et al., 2018). Wellness management of our stress responses, particularly to intergenerational and community-wide stresses that represent historical and ongoing trauma, can shift the response trajectory from negative to a balanced promotion of wellness and resilience. Importantly, earlier introduction of resilience factors enhances protection from "downstream" disease. For instance, while downstream recovery interventions such as pharmaceuticals, counselling, and land-based healing can be potentially restorative, they may be difficult to obtain and costly to implement. Furthermore, like secondary and tertiary prevention, downstream recovery interventions may not be fully effective and may be unable to undo years of sequelae. Resilient strategies (e.g., ceremony, spirituality, positive identity, holistic wellness), which come earlier and are preventive, can maintain balance

Figure 6.3. Trauma-based, resilience-informed model of Indigenous health

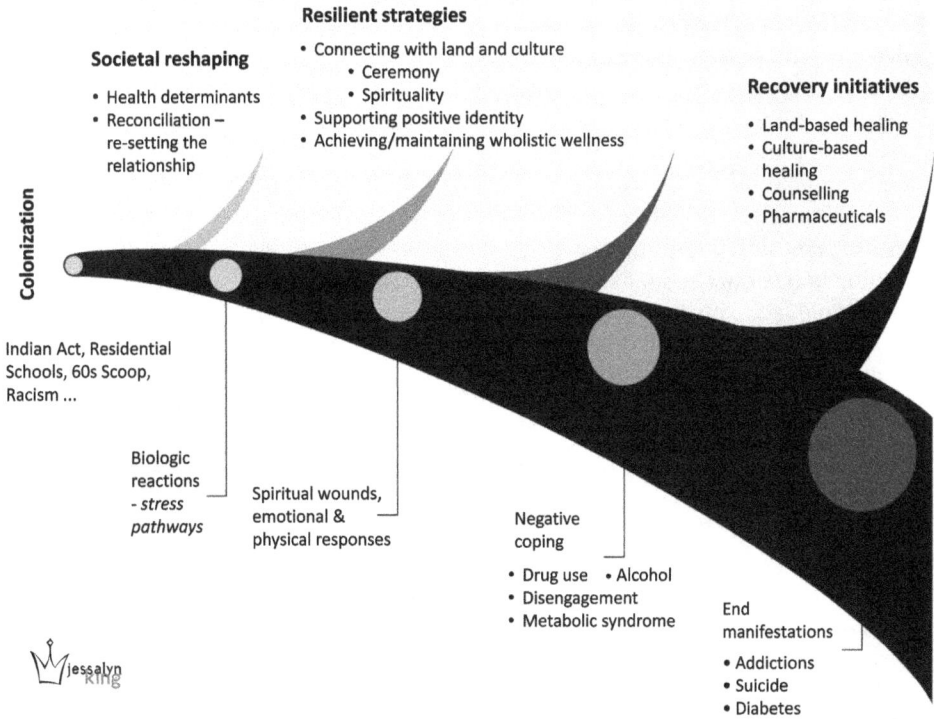

Resilient strategies
- Connecting with land and culture
  - Ceremony
  - Spirituality
- Supporting positive identity
- Achieving/maintaining wholistic wellness

Societal reshaping
- Health determinants
- Reconciliation – re-setting the relationship

Recovery initiatives
- Land-based healing
- Culture-based healing
- Counselling
- Pharmaceuticals

Colonization

Indian Act, Residential Schools, 60s Scoop, Racism ...

Biologic reactions - *stress pathways*

Spiritual wounds, emotional & physical responses

Negative coping
- Drug use   • Alcohol
- Disengagement
- Metabolic syndrome

End manifestations
- Addictions
- Suicide
- Diabetes

jessalyn King

Source: Dr. M. King.

and wellness. Not only are these strategies potentially cost-effective, but they are also protective against a broad range of end-manifestations. Ultimately, societal interventions dealing with Indigenous health determinants and addressing fundamental societal relationships (reconciliation) are critical in order to achieve health equity and to restore wellness for Indigenous peoples and Canadian society (Fayed et al., 2018).

Model projects will be shared that include Indigenous adolescents as partners; and connections with Elders, community leaders, and academic partners. The projects utilize principles of engagement and participatory action. These sample projects demonstrate the use of wise practice in the engagement of Indigenous youth functioning in collaboration with others to respond to challenges associated with diverse health concerns and conditions.

Resilient Strategies – Achieving/Maintaining Wellness

Brave Heart et al. (2011), Currie et al. (2012), and Paradies et al. (2013) described models of deterioration of Indigenous health due to exposure to trauma. Although the starting point could be racism, social exclusion, residential schools, or the removal of children from their homes, the models are fundamentally based on the trauma arising from colonization. Historical, ongoing, intergenerational traumas of colonization and post-colonial policies and practices lead to biological reactions (stresses), which then lead to emotional and physical responses, which in turn lead to negative coping behaviours and pathologies, ultimately leading to physical, mental, emotional, and spiritual end-manifestations (see figure 6.3).

The following section describes two projects that involve working with Indigenous youth that could serve as models for health research. Both projects involve working with Indigenous adolescents as partners and connecting them with Elders, community leaders, and academic partners to develop strategies to address health and wellness issues relevant to Indigenous youth goals.

1. *Indigenous Youth Mentorship: Diabetes. Deepening the roots of living in a good way for Indigenous Children – The Indigenous Youth Mentorship Program* (scientific lead, Dr. Jon McGavock, University of Manitoba) (CIHR, 2018).

Type 2 diabetes and obesity disproportionately affect Indigenous children and youth in Canada. Inequities in diabetes and obesity can be traced back to the transgenerational trauma, stress, and adversity that accompanies the ongoing institutional racism faced by Indigenous children and adolescents. Strengths-based, resilience-centred programs are therefore needed to overcome these inequities. With the support of Indigenous youth in Manitoba, the Pathways team developed a peer-based mentoring program, centred on an Indigenous model of resilience – Dr. Martin Brokenleg's Circle of Courage – called the Indigenous Youth Mentorship Program (see program website: www.jonmcgavock .com/aymp).

From a CIHR Pathways 2 Implementation funded research project, the team expanded from five communities in Manitoba to thirteen communities across four provinces in Canada. Using a participatory action model, guided by the teachings of Elders, knowledge holders, and youth on the team, this program is building on its successes to: (1) explore a novel pathway through which the Indigenous Youth Mentorship Program can reduce the risk of type 2 diabetes in youth through the Indigenous concept of *miyo-pimatisiwin*, "living in a good way"; (2) deepen the reach of this program within existing communities; (3) explore relational models of rippling the Indigenous Youth Mentorship Program to new communities; and (4) study the process of moving the Indigenous Youth Mentorship Program from a university-based program to a sustainable community-led organization. The outcomes of these studies will provide information and infrastructure to support rippling of other wellness-promoting community-based programs.

2. *The Healthy Sexuality Model*. *CheckUp: Time to focus on and learning from Inuit* (scientific lead, Dr. Alexandra King, University of Saskatchewan) (CIHR, 2017).

The CheckUp project is conducted with Inuit youth from Nunavik and Inuvialuit Region. Set in a context of concerns about sexually transmitted and blood-borne diseases among Inuit youth, the goals of the research are to: (1) normalize testing by changing attitudes and social norms around the use of screening services for sexually transmitted infections and other blood-borne infections, and reduce barriers to testing and linkage to care through streamlined pathways and innovative technologies; (2) decrease the burden of sexually transmitted infections and other blood-borne infections throughout Inuit Nunangat; (3) improve wellness and resiliency of Inuit youth using land-based and culture-based methods; (4) contextualize the CheckUp project in other Inuit regions; (5) foster Inuit youth leadership in planning of holistic health promotion interventions; and (6) elucidate an Inuit-derived Two-eyed Seeing approach to research and evaluation, employing both typical Western as well as Indigenous metrics, and ascertaining Inuit needs and methodologies.

CheckUp is following an implementation/program science approach (Becker et al., 2018) to advance and build on the effectiveness of early findings, emphasizing how interventions can be adapted to target other Inuit populations. The CheckUp team will examine what components of the project work best to influence change and how these components can be contextualized to communities in other Inuit regions. This process of contextualization will interweave the specific needs of each community, while building upon each community's strengths and unique ways of knowing and doing. Gender will be a particular focus of this project, replacing dichotomous or binary conceptualizations of gender with the much more diverse ones embraced by Indigenous peoples. Inuit-specific gender conceptualizations are an integral part of healthy sexuality and overall community wellness.

In sum, these two model projects involve working with Indigenous adolescents as partners, and connecting with Elders, community leaders, and academic partners in developing strategies to address health and wellness issues relevant to Indigenous youth goals. The projects follow principles of engagement and participatory action, and as such, have potential applicability to youth in other societies (such as immigrant/ newcomer youth and Indigenous youth in other countries), whose historical, social, cultural, or political contexts have led to disparities or vulnerabilities in health. These and similar projects serve as examples of wise practice in engagement for Indigenous youth working in partnership with others to address challenges linked to various health conditions or issues.

Conclusions

As research about Indigenous health in Canada expands from type 2 diabetes, mental illnesses and addictions, and sexually transmitted and blood-borne infections to a variety of other conditions, including respiratory health, the evidence regarding poorer health outcomes and inequitable access to care experienced by First Nations, Inuit, and Métis relative to non-Indigenous populations also expands. There is an increased understanding of how to work best with Indigenous peoples using robust frameworks operationalized in diverse contexts. These frameworks include Ethical Space, Two-eyed Seeing, and resilient strategies, which all privilege Indigenous ways of knowing and doing. Other critical guidelines involve collaboration with the relevant community in true partnership. Working with First Nations, Inuit, and Métis youth similarly requires respectful partnerships and strengths-based strategies that privilege Indigenous knowledge, while incorporating appropriate Western methods in culturally safe and responsive ways. This chapter also explored two exemplars of wellness-oriented implementation research and interventions, which emphasize upstream health determinants including connectivity to culture, language, and land; restoration of positive Indigeneity; and self-determination.

7 Supporting Refugee Adolescents

MIRIAM J. STEWART AND JOCELYN EDEY

Support Deficits for Refugees

Canada has been one of the top refugee destinations worldwide for hundreds of years (Government of Canada, 2018c). From 2000 to the second quarter of 2016, Canada welcomed over half a million refugees (Citizenship & Immigration Canada [CIC], 2016). From November 2015 to August 2018, Canada received more than 58,500 Syrian refugees (Government of Canada, 2018d). Our intervention study, completed in 2019, was influenced by recent humanitarian problems in Syria and focused on social support for refugee adolescents from Syria.

For youth, migration to a new country increases the risk of social problems such as isolation, service gaps, and support deficiencies. Newcomer youth's adaptation struggles are exacerbated by language obstacles and feelings of maginalization (Chrismas & Chrismas, 2017). Refugee youth and their families can experience stressors and traumatic events because of their migration, resettlement, and acculturation challenges (Pieloch et al., 2016). Empirical evidence has revealed acculturation problems that include unemployment, discrimination, and poverty among refugees (CIC, 2009; Community Foundation of Canada, 2010; Hou et al., 2016). Refugees can be targets of discrimination because of visible social markers such as skin colour, as well as cultural and religious traditions, which influence newcomers' health (Pocock & Chan, 2018; Szaflarski & Bauldry, 2019). Often refugees experience the loss of home and family members, and exposure to violence and torture (Jaranson et al., 2004). Intergenerational conflicts, financial constraints, employment struggles, inadequate knowledge about resources, language difficulties, and lack of transportation significantly impede newcomers' ability to mobilize or use supportive resources (M. Stewart, Anderson et al., 2008; Grewal et al., 2008). Refugees experience trauma when they are forced to seek refuge, leave their country in haste, and disrupt the parents' occupations and the children's education (Chrismas & Chrismas, 2017). Our previous research revealed that refugees experience greater support deficiencies than non-refugee immigrants (M. Stewart, Simich et al., 2011; M. Stewart, Simich et al., 2012; M. Stewart, Shizha et al., 2011). Migration, with family separation and detainment, and attendant lack of support from extended kin, may compromise the adaptation of refugee youth and their families (Mayo, 2018; Schweitzer et al., 2006; Warner, 2007).

As refugee families continue to come to Canada to escape persecution in their home countries, services must be created and modified, and policies and programs must be developed to foster successful adaptation (Hadfield et al., 2017). This chapter will illustrate how refugee adolescents can be supported to help both themselves and their peers adapt successfully and learn how to be resilient. The examination of a program designed to support the well-being of Syrian adolescent refugees may not only benefit this particular vulnerable population but also other groups of adolescents vulnerable to risks, stressors, and barriers to health. Accordingly, the aims of this chapter are twofold: to share insights from a study that designed and tested the social and cultural impacts of accessible, technology-based peer-support intervention for refugee adolescents from Syria; and to identify implications for programs, practice, and policies in social, health, and related sectors.

New strategies for supporting refugee youth are timely. Research has highlighted the potential beneficial effects of social support in buffering the stressful impacts of social isolation and adapting to a new culture (Simich et al., 2010; Uchida et al., 2008). Canadian policy documents revealed major challenges posing risks for refugee adolescents, and deficits in cultural appropriateness and accessibility of services and supports (Beiser et al., 2011; Bronstein & Montgomery, 2011; Fazel & Stein, 2002; Kirmayer et al., 2011; Oxman-Martinez et al., 2012; Simich et al., 2005;). Knowledge of the perceptions and experiences of refugee adolescents is deficient despite their unique challenges related to migration, settlement and integration, as well as developmental stressors (Edge et al., 2014).

Although support from peers and professionals is important for refugee adolescents and their families, our review revealed gaps in prior research regarding refugee youth intervention preferences and use of technology to enhance accessibility. Successful social support interventions focus on factors that promote social inclusion (e.g., shared language) and are culturally sensitive. Peer mentors who share the same culture, language, gender, and age, which can enhance shared experiential knowledge, are key to peer-support interventions. This shared knowledge and cultural suitability can improve utilization of support services. Emerging research has demonstrated that meeting refugee needs through peer programs that are culturally competent and sensitive appears to shorten the refugee transition period and make the transition less traumatic (Mitschke et al., 2017).

Culturally Sensitive Support Intervention

From 2005 to 2018, many refugees migrated to Western, Central, and Eastern Canada (e.g., 188,650 to Ontario, 37,114 to Alberta, and 4,179 to New Brunswick; Government of Canada, 2018a). The distribution of Syrian refugees since August 2018 included 2,670 in Edmonton, 1,565 in Windsor, and 610 in Fredericton (Government of Canada, 2018d). Adolescent refugees from Syria were recruited in these three Canadian cities. Reaching out to refugee adolescents during their initial years of arrival in Canada is timely (Guruge & Butt, 2015), as this is a particularly vulnerable time following migration. Refugees from Syria were recruited following consultations with collaborative agencies across Canada, including the Canadian Council of Refugees, Ontario Coalition of Agencies Serving Immigrants, Alberta Association of Immigrant Serving Agencies, New Brunswick Multicultural Council, and Saskatchewan Association of Immigrant Settlement and Integration Agencies.

Successful recruitment strategies used previously in our studies with immigrants and refugees, such as newcomer community organization staff and flyers in accessible languages (e.g., M. Stewart, Simich et al., 2011; M. Stewart, Simich et al., 2012; M. Stewart, Shizha et al., 2011), were used once again. Fifty Syrian adolescent refugees (24 female, 26 male) participated in this pilot intervention study. Participants were aged 13–19 years (25 aged 13–15 years, 25 aged 16–19 years), were recent refugees or refugee claimants, and had lived in Canada for less than two years.

The support intervention included four main features: (1) peer mentors and professional mentors; (2) provision and exchange of information, affirmation, and emotional support; (3) accessibility (bridge geographical boundaries, common language); and (4) groups comprised of like-gender and age-appropriate peers (young teens or older adolescents). Online support groups had ten to fifteen participants. Each group was co-led by a peer mentor who spoke both English and Arabic and was a former refugee from Syria (two male and two female peer mentors), and by a professional mentor (one male and one female). Peer mentors' experiential, first-hand knowledge of life as a refugee supplemented and complemented the knowledge of the professional mentor. Peer mentors demonstrated expertise in providing support, communicating, and coping with migration. Professional mentors had knowledge and work experience relevant to the challenges and support needs of Syrian refugee adolescents, social and health services for newcomers, and support programs. Peer mentors used their personal experiences to help participants feel comfortable sharing their own stories. The professionals provided support to the peer mentors regarding group process, technical challenges, and other issues.

Peer mentors participated in training sessions focused on support skills and online mentoring skills. A guide providing information about relevant topics and resources for support-group sessions was also developed for mentors. Weekly check-in meetings for peer and professional mentors were conducted to provide feedback, monitor progress, reassess strategies, and problem solve. Mentors stayed online after each support-group session to discuss successful strategies, changes for the next session, group dynamics, group members' interest in the session, and so on. The intervention provided a secure and reliable online meeting platform (GoToMeeting©) that enabled participants across the country to meet together with their peer mentor, professional mentor, and other Syrian refugee teens.

To ensure access to this technology-based support intervention, Chromebook PCs equipped with internet access were provided to participants who lacked computers with internet availability (twenty of fifty Syrian teen participants). Participant training in social networking technology and the internet was provided prior to the first support-group session. The initial session was conducted at accessible community sites (e.g., multicultural associations) to practise using the technology; meet fellow participants and mentors; select preferred discussion topics; and introduce the participant orientation handbook.

To avoid language barriers, support groups were conducted in the language of choice of the majority of participants, English or Arabic. Most group sessions were held in Arabic. In addition, youth in each group chose optimum times for support sessions so that work, school, and family obligations would not be obstacles to participation.

Discussion topics were informed by our teams' previous research with over 200 non-refugee adolescents and with more than 150 refugee parents of adolescents. Topics included issues related to school, friendships, family separation, family relationships, rights, cultural conflict, conflict resolution, social isolation, social exclusion, cultural adaptation, citizenship and immigration, education, social activities, community resources, resource access, support seeking, and coping strategies. All PowerPoint slides and support intervention documents were translated from English to Arabic.

Peer and professional mentors selected appropriate support and educational materials to augment online program content, based on adolescent participants' preferences. Participants shared their computer screen to show art, view PowerPoint presentations, interact on-screen, and chat online with other group members across sites. PowerPoint slides were tailored to be appealing and appropriate in terms of culture, language, gender, and age. Content experts familiar with peer-support programs and research staff with knowledge of the language and culture of participants were consulted in program development. Participants had the opportunity to explore a range of game options appealing in terms of age, gender, interests, ethnicity, and culture, which facilitated interactions with peers. Drawing tools, highlighters, graphics, online videos, and reading materials were used as facilitation aids to enhance relevance and appeal of the online program.

To maximize the sustainable effects of the support program and optimize age-appropriate duration and frequency, the social-support intervention was conducted over eight sessions, weekly or biweekly (dependent on group participant preferences and availability). Sessions lasted approximately sixty to ninety minutes. Participants chose whether and how they would connect with each other (e.g., telephone, email) between online group sessions. Participants could also seek or accept interim support from peer or professional mentors by phone, text, or email.

Evaluation of the Online Support Program

A mixed-methods design, using both qualitative and quantitative methods, was employed in this study. Standardized quantitative measures were administered at two points (pre-test and post-test) to determine outcomes of the support intervention. Again, to ensure accessibility in terms of literacy and language, questionnaires and interview guides were administered by research assistants in either Arabic or English, depending on participant preferences. Pre-test standardized quantitative measures of coping, loneliness, social support, post-traumatic stress, and social connectedness were completed with fifty Syrian adolescents prior to the intervention, and post-test measures were completed with forty-six participants at the conclusion of the intervention (92 per cent response rate).

Through qualitative methods (Dam et al., 2017), we gained in-depth insight into refugee adolescent experiences, support satisfaction, and intervention process. An eight-item semi-structured interview guide included questions about participants' satisfaction with the intervention online format and tools; perceived intervention impacts; suggestions for change; social interaction during support-group sessions; communication with other participants or peer/professional mentors between the online group sessions; and continued contacts with other participants. Thirty-four (68 per cent) of the teens participated in post-intervention group interviews (10 males and 13 females) or individual interviews (5 males and 6 females) based on participant preferences. Interviews were conducted in Arabic, transcribed, and translated into English.

Post-intervention individual interviews were also conducted with all peer mentors in their language of choice, using a ten-item semi-structured interview guide that elicited information regarding mentor roles, co-leadership with professional mentors, perceived intervention impacts, and recommended changes. After each online support-group session, peer mentors completed field notes to document the types of support provided and exchanged; topics discussed during the group sessions; group process; and out-of-session contacts with participants. Professional mentors provided written responses to ten questions following completion of the intervention, which focused on both intervention processes and impacts.

Syrian Youths' Initial Experiences in Canada

During online support-group sessions, teen participants began by discussing their initial experiences in Canada. Refugee adolescents primarily discussed how, where, and what type of help they received when they first arrived in Canada. Sources of help included other students, teachers, and members of the local community. "I think the Canadian society is a very helpful society. People in Canadian society help even if you don't know someone a lot" (male, older youth). "I am feeling that people are so helpful even if I don't have the [English] language" (female, older youth). One participant described feeling lost, both figuratively and literally, and needing help: "I felt lost because everything around me was new ... I would go to places and get lost ... then things became normal" (male, older youth). Most participants described immigration challenges stemming from language barriers. "We found difficulties in language and culture and we have to communicate with others and how to express our ideas. As you know the language is the key and it is really hard for us" (female, older youth). "My school experience was difficult at the beginning, because we didn't know the language" (male, older youth).

As a female adolescent refugee explained, Syrian refugees perceived everything in Canada as different: "Everything was different ... from my country and [I had] difficulties with everything." Difficulties with differences included: the English language, school, Canadian culture, the weather, food, and focus on time. An older male youth described the "time" challenge: "Everything was timed and there was nothing you could do about it. We were not used to that routine; everything is tied to time. Everything goes according to time here in Canada."

Participants described the Canadian school system as positively different from the Syrian system. School in Canada was perceived as less stressful, more focused on preparation, with more choice of future study topics, and less-strict discipline: "In Syria, they beat students as a way of disciplining them, so they use sticks to beat students. However, in Canada they respect students. Here in Canada they don't use violence to discipline students" (male, young youth).

Participants also noted cultural differences between Syria and Canada. They highlighted the multicultural nature of the Canadian culture. A male peer mentor explained:

What I love in Canada is that there is multiculturalism. So here there is no one particular culture ... So, because of multiculturalism in Canada when you come here as a fresh person you feel like you are one of the different people already here. That is really nice, because you feel like you are one of them, you feel like you are integrated already. You feel like you can engage people. You don't feel like you are alone, you don't feel that you are different. And that helps a lot.

Freedom and diversity were identified as benefits of living in Canada by many participants.

In Canada there is individual freedom, and everyone can talk to anyone, including girls, without restrictions. (Male, older youth).

It is really nice as a community here ... [there is] huge diversity and being here gave us a chance to know more people. For example, yesterday was Chinese New Year and that was the first time to hear about it. So that is really nice to know about other's cultures and interests. It is really nice that we all respect each other. (Female, young youth)

Nobody cares what you wear. Maybe someone doesn't like what you wear, but nobody comments on [this]. (Male, older youth)

Differences between Canada and Syria also included having fewer friends and feeling isolated and alone:

> In school I was feeling strange and lonely in the first year, because I knew nobody and had no friends in the school. (Male, young youth)
>
> I felt we were alone; no language and it was really difficult ... I had a hard time finding friends ... but then everything has changed. When I got to school, I learned the English language faster and life became easier. I felt at the beginning it was really hard and I was telling my dad that I wanted to go back to home country. (Female, older youth)

Syrian Youths' Experiences in Intervention

Participants described the support they received prior to and during the online peer-support program. Most adolescents indicated that their parents strongly encouraged them to join the program and to continue participation. Parents advised their children that the program would be a great opportunity. Cited benefits included making new friends, learning from others, talking with people, learning more English, and learning about Canada. A young male adolescent participant explained that he was shy and stayed home prior to the program. When his parents heard about the online support intervention, they "encouraged me to attend the program to meet people I didn't know and to learn to talk with people I didn't know."

Four key processes were revealed in this intervention program. The first process was *building relationships*. This encompassed the importance of meeting new people and making new friendships: "The program helped me to deepen my friendships with friends I knew already and in being able to talk with more confidence to people I didn't know before. The program helped me to not be afraid of talking to people I don't know" (male, young adolescent). Relationships were key to helping participants feel less isolated during and following the intervention program. Terms such as "community," "team," and "friends" were used to explain how teens felt less alone as a result of this support program:

> Before the online program, participants were not communicating with or talking much to each other. Everyone was keeping in their homes and didn't have many friends or much contact with others. After we joined the program, we became connected and we continue to connect ... I felt I was not alone. I felt I have friends not only from the city where I live, but friends from other parts of Canada. I felt like I am part of a group that is one team. (Female, older youth)

Improved communication skills had numerous positive impacts: "It made life easier and helped me to be more social and talk to people" (female, young adolescent). The following quote from a young Syrian female demonstrates how relationships and shared experiences were intertwined:

> You feel like you are lonely; that you can't express yourself, you feel like you don't have friends. After you join the program, you begin to make friends, you begin to tell them about yourself, you have an incredible opportunity for people to discover who you are, you begin to express yourself, and people begin to treat you the right way and you begin to have confidence in yourself, and you feel like you are not alone anymore. (Female, young youth)

Sharing facilitated the building of relationships. "What I liked best was being able to talk and connect with Syrian youths in Canada I didn't know before" (male, young youth). Another youth said, "We all are communicating together and know more friends ... this program was really nice and helped me to be more confident and [overcome] the challenge that I was so shy and not brave to talk to people, but now it really changed my personality" (female, young youth). An older female youth said, "I like it so much because usually I am not a social person, but this program made me more engaged." A young female teen explained how she would recommend this program to a friend: "... you will meet new people and know new experiences and new stories about people. This will help a lot to know more about a new country ... Peoples' experiences are the most important thing to learn from."

A peer mentor clarified that through relationships and shared experiences, participants "used weaknesses to become strong." A young female participant described how the program helped create new relationships: "Knowing new people will help me to be more engaged and to love my life ... It helps me to know more people from my community and to know that I am not by myself, and there are other people going through difficulties that I am going through."

When asked how they would describe this program to a friend, participants said they would explain how it offers an opportunity to meet new people, make friends, be part of a community, and share experiences.

The second process was *sharing experiences*. Through the sharing of experiences, Syrian youth built relationships with people they did not know and with some that they already did know, allowing them to learn from each other. "It was an opportunity for Syrian participants ... to talk about themselves and to share what they liked, what they didn't, what their dreams are, and what careers they would like to pursue in the future" (female, young youth). Sharing experiences was the most valued component of this support intervention program. "It gave me an opportunity to build something like a community of friends" (male, older youth). Another explained:

> It was a nice group to be part of and what I liked most is how each partici-
> pant was talking about the experiences they have been through, so I felt
> that we have the same problems, struggles, and how they get through it ... I
> felt more hopeful to do more things and I can do whatever I want and noth-
> ing is impossible. (Female, young youth)

Participants shared family dreams and life stories, experiences, views, history, challenges, goals, and difficulties. Peer mentors reported that Syrian adolescent participants compared challenges (e.g., new culture, language) and shared coping strategies. These mentors described their role during support-group sessions as encouraging participants to respect, listen, and share their experiences, dreams, and challenges.

The third process was *learning*. Peer mentors reported that participants learned from each other, and from both peer and professional mentors. Participants learned persistence, leadership, optimism, and resilience; and they learned how to overcome difficult experiences, view challenges through different perspectives, be positive, find people to trust, and learn from others' mistakes. One older female adolescent said, "The online support program was a great step in helping Syrian participants, as newcomers to Canada, learn about things that are helpful in their daily life in Canada. Sharing experiences and exchange of ideas and communication between participants was useful because it allowed them to learn from each other."

Peer mentors believed that learning led to participants gaining new capabilities and confidence. Learning about the option of going to school *and* working at the same time was intriguing to these Syrian teens, who had not previously considered this as a possiblity. This helped youth plan to pursue an advanced degree while finishing secondary school. Learning how to communicate with others and learning about life in Canada were considered advantageous parts of this program.

> I learned a lot from the youths who shared their experiences during the
> sessions. Listening to youth share their experience and engaging in discus-
> sions in the group helped me learn things I didn't know before and were
> helpful to me ... the benefit I got from participating in the program might
> be [considered] little, but in the end it made a huge difference for me.
> (Male, older adolescent)

Participants reported learning many important things: English language, where to seek help, how to overcome challenges, and other "things you didn't know." Professional and peer mentors described Syrian youth as "open to learning."

The fourth process was *seeking support.* Participants reported that they learned how and where to access support from community members, service organizations, teachers, family members, and peers.

> I didn't do a lot of things before I joined the program. I didn't know how to ask for help. I didn't know who was supposed to help me with my school challenges. I didn't know how to talk to people. After I joined the program, I began to be able to talk to people and to make friends. I was then able to make friends who helped me with school challenges that I sometimes faced. (Male, older youth)

These four processes in Syrian teens' experiences in the peer support-education program are interconnected. As relationships are created, trust is built, resulting in the sharing of experiences. This supports refugee youth as they learn new information and coping skills that enhance their lives.

Program Content and Support

Many participants reported that the sessions focused on planning and goals for the future were most beneficial. To illustrate, one older female youth described the sessions' content: "The topics that talked about how to succeed in life, steps to success, time management, how to plan for the future, and supports available whether from school, organizations, and in the community." These Syrian youth articulated their individual goals and then explored ways to achieve them. As a Syrian female peer mentor explained:

> Those sessions gave participants an impression about goals, because at the beginning they sounded like they were lost. Even if the participants are attending school, they may have different ideas in their minds about goals. Most of the participants didn't come here directly from Syria. Most of them came to Canada from other countries like Jordan, so they might have made friends in those places and being in all those different places might have made things a little blurred in their minds. So the sessions around goals helped the participants to have a plan. A plan like how to start, how to be clear in your goals and in setting your goals, how to get the right support from the right people, and to be engaged in the

community. So I felt those sessions around goals and goal setting helped the participants a lot.

In these sessions, Syrian teen participants talked about realizing their dreams and goals, Canadian culture, Canadian weather, school systems in Canada, and concurrent work and study.

Participants described peer and professional mentors as encouraging, motivating, inspiring, and capable. Peer mentors clarified that the primary source of support provided to participants was emotional support, which started with helping refugee youth feel safe and comfortable, listening, and encouraging. This facilitated the delivery of the online intervention program. Professional mentors also provided varied supports, such as clarifying content, helping with homework, solving technology issues, encouraging friendships, advising, sharing, and communicating. Both peer and professional mentors provided support for overcoming language barriers through translation, as one professional mentor described:

> What went well was also the strategy of allowing participants to feel free to speak in a language they felt comfortable speaking: English or Arabic. So, there were no challenges with participants communicating what they wanted to say, as far as language is concerned, because they had the choice to speak Arabic or English.

A male peer mentor explained that participants found it easier to communicate in Arabic, which "gave them the encouragement to share their experiences with ease."

Most teen participants described the different ways they connected with their peers during and following the program. Some Syrian adolescents who lived in the same city connected in person, which helped to transform acquaintances into friends: "I got closer in my friendships with the participants from my city ... I now meet and talk everyday with these friends, which was not the case before I joined the program ... So I don't feel lonely anymore" (male, young adolescent).

Participants also reported using social media to stay connected to their friends in the support group during the program. Facebook and WhatsApp were identified as the most common tools for online communication: "I got connected with participants on WhatsApp and I was always [communicating] with these friends, where we talked about everything ... WhatsApp group helped me feel less lonely" (male, older adolescent). Participants described talking about the program, how to overcome challenges, life in Canada, language difficulties, and the future. "We talked about how amazing the online program was, and the opportunity it gave the participants to share their experiences. We became friends and stayed in touch" (female, young adolescent). Relationship building and networking was beneficial for diminishing loneliness and maintaining a sense of community for refugee adolescents who were scattered across Canada.

Interpretation of Intervention

Three social processes – social exchange, social comparison, social learning – inform interpretation of this support intervention (Borkman; 1999; David, 1999; Molm, 1997). As close relationships developed between refugee participants and their peer supporters, reciprocity and *social exchange* became evident in their interactions. Participants exchanged strategies to meet people they did not know previously, cope with challenges, speak better English, and ask for help. According to *social comparison* theory, individuals compare themselves and affiliate with others (e.g., peers in groups with a shared language and culture) who have first-hand experiential knowledge of a stressful situation. Participants explained the value of creating a community with peers who share the common experience of being a Syrian adolescent refugee, speaking Arabic, and facing similar challenges and difficulties. This peer support, based on first-hand "experiential knowledge," is a critical source of *social learning* for vulnerable refugees and can supplement professional knowledge.

Impacts of Intervention on Syrian Refugee Youth

Many Syrian refugee teens reported decreased isolation and loneliness; increased self-confidence; enhanced knowledge of available information, opportunities, and resources for refugees; as well as improved coping strategies. Youth participants felt more optimistic about their ability to handle challenges, as well as their opportunities and future in Canada. One professional mentor reported that they saw significant improvement in participants' understanding of life in Canada, how to build strategies to succeed in school and life, how to seek support, and how to cope with challenges. A male peer mentor maintained that this program could have a positive impact on future Syrian refugees:

> The refugee community benefited in that the participants gained new ideas and new experiences through their participation in the online program. So, the Syrian refugee community will be in a position to advise new Syrian refugees that will arrive in Canada, because they will have been in Canada for three or more years and they will have experience of life in Canada.

The most common way this online support program helped Syrian teens to cope with challenges was teaching them how to seek support:

> I didn't know how to cope with problems before. The online support program helped me understand that it's okay to ask for help and I came to realize that the help I need ... is available if I ask for it ... It's a very useful program. You get to know Syrian youth from other parts of Canada. You learn from their experiences; you get to know what types of help you can get to deal with your challenges and problems. (Male, young Syrian youth)

Learning how to overcome challenges and cope with problems was an important program outcome:

> Before I joined the program ... I didn't know how to deal with challenges ... After I joined the program, I became more confident ... I discovered that I could actually get help from people beyond school that could help with not only school challenges and problems, but with anything. The program helped me understand that if I have a problem or challenge, I can get help to solve it not only from my school teacher but from a variety of people and organizations in the community. (Young female Syrian teen)

Syrian youth reported that the online support program was useful, positive, exciting, and informative. A Syrian peer mentor clarified why the program succeeded:

> I felt the participants needed somebody they can look up to: somebody who can open their heart and arms to, and give them a little time to hear and listen to what they are saying and thinking; and to lead them the right way; and to make them feel that they have someone to mentor or coach them, to help them.

The impacts of the intervention on social isolation, support-seeking coping, social networks, perceived trauma, and social connectedness outcomes were assessed using both qualitative and quantitative methods. These impacts were described above in the qualitative data summary. Quantitative survey results revealed similar positive impacts. A paired-samples t-test of participants' pre- and post-test intervention scores indicated an increase in perceived social support. The overall mean score of 69 ($SD = 10.5$) rose to 73.2 [($SD = 7.37$); $t(40) = -2.36, p = 0.02$] following the support intervention. This increase in perceived support was statistically significant. Moreover, quantitative results revealed positive trends in increased social connectedness, improved coping, and decreased loneliness after participation in the intervention (although non-statistically significant).

Implications for Refugee Adolescent Programs

Youth newcomers to Canada often experience s*ocial isolation* (Amthor & Roxas, 2016), which can be an obstacle to accessing formal support services (Shields & Lujan, 2018), a barrier that can carry over to succeeding generations (Banulescu-Bogdan, 2020). The Syrian youth refugees in this study frequently described feelings of loneliness. These newcomers often stayed at home because of meager social contacts and insufficient knowledge about how or where to seek support. After participating in this program, participants reported feeling less alone and more part of a team. Syrian teens learned that it is acceptable to ask for help. Talking to peers and learning from each other built friendships and connections that helped them adjust to life in Canada.

Given cultural differences around seeking support, the significance of supportive resources aimed at specific needs of refugees is critical. Supportive persons can alter the appraisal of stressors, sustain coping efforts, and influence the choice of coping strategies (Gottlieb, 2000). Common coping skills used by young African refugees, in a previous study, focused on hope for the future (Gladden, 2012). Similarly, young Syrian refugees in our study expressed the value of planning for their future and learning strategies to achieve their goals.

Professional mentors noted positive implications of this online support intervention for programs and services targeting refugee youth. Participants felt "more optimistic now about their ability to deal with challenges they face, as well as about the opportunities and their future in Canada." They emphasized the importance of providing an opportunity for refugee youth to "chat freely" and compare their situation with other refugee adolescents. Providing information, support, and time to share experiences with peers is significant for the success of refugee youth programs.

When refugee adolescents offered suggestions for enhancing this intervention program, most emphasized technological issues. A few thought additional introductory computer skills would be useful as most participants did not initially have email accounts or computer operational knowledge (e.g., accessing websites, opening documents.). The research team provided computer and internet skills training for participants to help them use their computers/laptops; access their email; and open the link to use GoToMeeting© effectively. In Edmonton, the professional mentor visited homes to assist participants before the start of the program. In Fredericton, collaborators organized a training session at a local community centre with WiFi access that focused on creating accounts and use of the internet. Having a user-friendly online platform was considered essential. Program improvement suggestions also included increasing session length to allow more time for socializing, introductions, discussion of unplanned topics, and practising speaking English if desired.

Rich data were gleaned from these refugee youth. Participants were comfortable with the interviewer who was fluent in written and spoken Arabic, and experienced in conducting research and community programs with North African refugees and immigrants. Service organizations could select applicable content and processes from this support intervention, and adapt it for their own clients. Future programs could benefit from exploring other online platforms that are easily accessible and encompass document viewer capabilities, webinar functions, and networking features to foster relationships.

Refugees build a sense of belonging when they spend time in established groups of peers facing similar stressors related to adjustment in a new society. Online support interventions can improve accessibility to peer support in terms of time, physical constraints, and stigma related to professional help-seeking (Blom et al., 2013, 2014; Boots et al., 2014). Online support programs can also provide opportunities for anonymous interaction and information exchange (Dam et al., 2017). Our previous studies revealed that vulnerable adolescents and their parents wanted accessible technology-enabled support, such as online peer groups (Makwarimba et al., 2017; M. Stewart, Dennis et al., 2015; M. Stewart, Letourneau et al., 2013; M. Stewart, Simich et al., 2012; M. Stewart, Barnfather et al., 2011).

Although some refugee adolescent participants expressed problems coping, the resilience of refugee youth should be reinforced. Supporters and service providers are encouraged to emphasize refugee youths' strengths, recognize knowledge and capabilities obtained through previous experiences, acknowledge supports in refugee youths' own networks, and employ these resources to help refugee youth cope with challenges (Pieloch et al., 2016). Refugee youth arrive in new countries with "experiences and histories of loss, trauma, uncertainty, and upheaval" (Marshall et al., 2016, p. 316). Although their pre-migration and migration stressors place them at increased risk for mental health problems, they can settle into Canada with new skills, abilities, and hope (Marshall et al., 2016; Masten, 2012). Social support, a sense of belonging, valuing education, optimism, family connectedness, and cultural connections promote resilience for refugee youth (Pieloch et al., 2016). Opportunities to engage in their new country's culture enhances experiences of well-being (Berry & Hou, 2016). There is significant potential to elevate refugee adolescent well-being through cross-sector and interdisciplinary approaches, in which settlement, education, health, and numerous other sectors function collectively (Hadfield et al., 2017). Services should be culturally and linguistically customized, consistent with refugee preferred location and mode, and accessible (Khan, 2019). The intervention shared in this chapter has the potential to influence the support of the most vulnerable new members of Canadian society.

SECTION III

Parents' Experiences

Section III Introduction: Parents' Experiences

JOCELYN EDEY

This final section of the book transitions from direct lived experiences of children and adolescents to reciprocally linked experiences of parents/caregivers. Early childhood development is shaped by economic and social resources available to parents, and a child's health can influence the parents' socio-economic status. Demands on parents caring for a child with a chronic illness without sufficient support can negatively affect the parents' physical and mental well-being. The chapters in this section will investigate factors that influence the health of parents, innovative support programs to address their needs, and insights for relevant services.

Chapter 8, "Low-Income Parents and Caregivers of Children Affected by Health Challenges," will explore the helplessness, frustration, and fear of low-income parents, grandparents, and other family members caring for a child with health challenges. The cycle of poverty and health problems is examined as poor living conditions can exacerbate health problems that in turn diminish the family's limited resources and contribute to deteriorating living conditions. These parents experience stigma linked with poverty, guilt at their inability to provide for their children, and practical concerns associated with limited funds for costly medications, childcare, and an improved living environment. This chapter will also share a support-education program tailored for the needs of these vulnerable parents.

Next, chapter 9, "Indigenous Parents and Caregivers Caring for Children with Chronic Health Conditions," will examine a program designed to help parents of Indigenous children overcome obstacles as they struggle to provide optimal care. This Indigenous peer-support program was created in response to the unique cultural challenges identified in interviews with Indigenous parents and family caregivers of children with a chronic health condition. The chapter will describe how parents, who are frequently overwhelmed by poverty, must deal directly with health care and social service systems they distrust; battle discrimination; and navigate a culture that does not understand their unique needs. Building on research analyses of their complex challenges, this chapter highlights a support program designed to overcome barriers faced by Indigenous parents.

Chapter 10, "Innovative Programs for Parents Coping with Health Inequities: Informed by Research Insights," concludes this section with an exploration of programs designed to address the risk factors, needs, and strengths of four different groups of vulnerable parents: refugee new parents, mothers experiencing post-partum depression, mothers suffering with an abusive partner, and parents of children with respiratory problems. These programs will highlight transformative knowledge translation strategies designed and tested in paediatric and community health settings to improve outcomes for vulnerable parents, families, and the health system. The ultimate aim of these knowledge translation and transfer initiatives is to ensure that evidence from research-tested interventions is used in communities and health service facilities to enhance the health of vulnerable parents and children.

Social determinants of child and adolescent health include those to which their parents are exposed (Raphael, 2014). Diverse challenges and barriers face refugee parents, parents with post-partum depression, parents in abusive relationships, parents of children with chronic illness, as well as others who face stigma and isolation. Common challenges reported by vulnerable parents in the reported studies will highlight information gaps, geographical challenges, stigma, financial constraints, and culturally insensitive services. Reported benefits of support programs explored in this chapter include decreased isolation, marginalization and exclusion; enhanced inclusion and health literacy; and stakeholder engagement.

8 Low-Income Parents and Caregivers of Children Affected by Health Challenges

MIRIAM J. STEWART

Over 4 million (13 per cent) people in Canada are living on low incomes (Statistics Canada, 2018a). Many Canadians at risk of being low-income are living in a single-parent household. Forty-four per cent of female lone-parent families with children from birth to seventeen years of age are low-income. This percentage increases to 60.4 per cent when children are five years old and under (Statistics Canada, 2018a). Other groups at increased risk of being low-income are non-permanent residents, which include refugee claimants and their families (42.9 per cent) (Statistics Canada, 2016a), and self-identified Aboriginal people, one quarter of whom live in low-income circumstances (Statistics Canada, 2016b). Social investments, particularly for families with children living in poverty, are required to enhance health equity (Public Health Agency of Canada [PHAC], 2008).

In modern industrialized nations such as Canada, poverty poses a barrier that limits participation in cultural, economic, educational, political, and other societal activities. Poverty is a principal cause of disease, illness, and shortened life expectancy, which deeply affects Canadians' quality of life and the physical, psychological, emotional, and social health of individuals and families (Robinson, 2019). Income provides prerequisites for health, including housing, food, clothing, education, and safety. Poverty can restrict opportunities to achieve full health potential because it limits choices. People with limited access to income can experience social isolation, stress, inadequate housing, environmental pollution, and physical and mental health challenges, which in turn contribute to a downward spiral into poverty (Shimmin, 2015). The effects of exclusion on low-income Canadians' health and quality of life can be excessive (Raphael, 2006).

Health problems among low-income children are increased by income-related risk factors (e.g., environmental conditions), and children's health problems can, in turn, increase the family's risk of living in poverty (Lukemeyer et al., 2004). Indeed, low-income conditions can directly influence the symptoms and treatment of respiratory-related conditions. Socio-economic status is associated with more asthma exacerbations requiring urgent care (Ungar et al., 2011) and emergency room visits for low-income parents and families than for middle-to-upper-income families (Sin et al., 2003). Financial challenges create significant barriers to positive health outcomes. For example, many people cannot afford medication, and many insurance carriers do not provide complete coverage (Asthma Society of Canada, 2014).

This chapter will explore the perspectives of low-income parents, elicited in two nationally funded studies, who have children living with a chronic respiratory condition. The aim of this chapter is to present insights regarding parents' needs, circumstances, and preferences and to provide a glimpse into the lives of families coping with challenges of respiratory problems and with constraints of low-income. The insights of health and social service professionals are also shared to describe challenges faced by low-income parents and families. The perspectives of both parents and service providers/program planners that are described in this chapter are critical to informing the creation of an equitable and accessible support program.

Low-Income Parents' Perspectives and Preferences

Support Gaps and Stressors Faced by Parents

Low-income parents were asked about their available support services, support gaps, and program preferences. Purposive sampling was used (M. Stewart, Masuda et al., 2015) to identify potential participants representing varied low-income situations (e.g., working poor, social assistance recipients, unemployed, homeless) and key demographic characteristics such as gender, ethnicity, immigration status, and age that may influence low-income status. Participants were recruited through community service agencies, community networks, child clinics, and voluntary organizations serving low-income people. Research staff distributed flyers and posters at community agencies, and recruitment notices were shared on family websites and at low-income schools and at a food bank. Draws for grocery gift cards were conducted at community sites and entrants were invited to participate in the study. The most effective recruitment tool was a flyer delivery to low-income housing complexes. Eligibility criteria for inclusion as study participants, in addition to low income, included being a parent/primary family caregiver of a child with respiratory health problems and having a level of comfort speaking English. The study sites were two large urban cities in Western Canada. Thirty-seven parents took part in this study (twenty-five from Edmonton, twelve from Winnipeg). Sixty-one per cent of the Edmonton families interviewed lived in low-income housing complexes and all Winnipeg families lived in subsidized housing. Almost one half of participants (49 per cent) represented ethnic groups, including Indigenous and immigrant peoples.

FINANCIAL STRESS

Living on a low income increased challenges of managing a child's respiratory condition, and respiratory conditions made living on a low income more challenging. Asthma contributed to the families' poverty through costs of medication, food, housing, and parents' underemployment or unemployment. Many parents had been laid off, worked part time, or chose self-employment because of health crises in their families, including spending time with their child at emergency departments and hospitals, or caring for a sick child at home. Self-employment allowed parents the flexibility to care for their children. However, their children's chronic respiratory condition limited the time the parents were available to work and promote their business. Since their incomes were variable, at times parents did not qualify for low-income pharmaceutical coverage. Some parents could not find affordable and safe childcare. Parents perceived that health professionals did not understand the difficulties inherent in managing the intertwined health, home, work, and community challenges made even more complex because of low incomes.

In Canada, the health care system is considered a national system but only covers a limited range of services (core medical and emergency services) at the point of care within different provincial and territorial funded plans. Accordingly, vulnerable populations have difficulties accessing necessary health care linked to long wait times for elective care, inequitable access to health services in both public and private systems, and lack of prescription medication coverage (Martin et al., 2018). According to the Government of Canada (2018e), the Canada Health Act provides, at no cost, prescription drugs administered in Canadian hospitals but, outside of the hospital setting, provincial and territorial governments are responsible for administration of publicly funded drug plans. The federal, provincial, and territorial governments offer varying levels of coverage. Overall the publicly funded drug programs provide drug plan coverage for those most in need, based on age, income, and medical condition. Many Canadians and their family members have drug coverage linked to employment, while some Canadians (e.g., adults aged eighteen to twenty-four or over sixty-five) have no drug coverage and pay the full cost of prescription drugs (Bolatova & Law, 2019; Government of Canada, 2018e).

This gap was reflected in parent-reported concerns about problems families face when their income slightly exceeds low-income cut-offs and costs of medications are no longer covered. Parents noted that private pharmaceutical coverage did not pay for asthma medication because it was a pre-existing condition. Additionally, even with private coverage, some parents had to pay out-of-pocket for co-pay or the entire medication bill and then wait for reimbursement. Some participants believed that rescue inhalers or less expensive controller medications were prescribed because of their poverty, and that their low-income status limited access to preventive medications and referrals to specialists. Some parents found costs of preventive medications hard to justify when symptoms did not seem severe, and when money was needed for other life expenses. Medications were sometimes rationed for emergency use to make them last longer or shared between children to reduce costs (M. Stewart, Masuda et al., 2015). Another salient study found that in 25 per cent of Canadian households, someone is not taking their medication because of their inability to pay (Angus Reid Institute, 2015). Parents were often forced to make difficult decisions due to limited finances, which caused severe stress, knowing that their children's special needs for food or medicine might be unmet. They explained that allergies could limit food choices, and safe foods like soy milk were expensive. Parents were also unable to afford health supplements, such as vitamins, that were important to their children's health.

CHILDCARE AND TRANSPORTATION CHALLENGES
Care for siblings in a health emergency or during medical appointments was a common challenge. Parents had to either find a sitter who could care for their other children or bring them with the sick child. Finding childcare for children with respiratory conditions was also challenging. Parents worried that childcare providers would not respond appropriately when their children were in respiratory distress, and some children were rejected from daycare centres, as staff did not feel adequately prepared to handle their health condition. Transportation was another barrier to accessing available resources. Walking or taking buses to medical appointments with ill children or finding funds for a taxi or ambulance in emergencies was a significant deterrent for most parents.

ENVIRONMENT AND EDUCATION BARRIERS

Although parents were aware of environmental triggers, they were frustrated by the lack of control over their living conditions. Many expressed concern about negative effects of housing on their children's health. Low-income families could not afford safe, healthy housing. Parents reported that they had not been informed about factors influencing their children's condition. For example, some physicians explained the condition; others just gave parents an inhaler. Only a few parents received referrals for asthma education from emergency clinics, after a child's hospitalization. They found education helpful in understanding their children's condition and care. One parent indicated that a pharmacist showed them how to administer the child's medication. Another parent noted that asthma education was offered, but at a prohibitive cost of a hundred and fifty dollars, "They told me that I had to pay up front and everything. When they turned me away, I just started crying."

DISCRIMINATORY HEALTH CARE INTERACTIONS

Parents described discrimination in their relationships with health and social service professionals. Low-income family caregivers reported non-supportive encounters with the health system. Health professionals questioned parents'/caregivers' judgment and knowledge of children's symptoms. Parents thought health service providers did not understand their difficulty managing the complex intertwined home, work, and community challenges associated with respiratory health conditions, which are complicated by low income. Indeed, parents felt blamed for being poor. Family caregivers, overwhelmed by perceived power differentials when dealing with service providers in health and health-related sectors, wanted reassurance that their children's respiratory problem was not their fault, and affirmation that they had the requisite skills and knowledge to manage (M. Stewart, Evans et al., 2016; M. Stewart, King et al., 2013).

SUPPORT PREFERENCES AND PROGRAMS

Parents were keenly interested in sharing their experiences with other low-income parents of children with respiratory health problems. They wanted to learn from these peers specific strategies for dealing with condition exacerbations and for finding cheaper medications and available resources. Parents also needed emotional support gained from talking to other parents in similar circumstances. Opportunities to share their personal experiences and learn from peers in-person was considered beneficial, but the accessibility of online support was also welcomed. Online support groups, delivered by peer mentors and by a health professional, were recommended. Parents contended that time, geographic location, distance, childcare for siblings, and lack of organizational support posed barriers to attending face-to-face support-education programs.

Low-Income Parent Support Intervention

The purpose of this follow-up study was to design and test a pilot program that provided support and education to low-income parents of children who have respiratory health conditions, using computer and telephone support. Participants were drawn from low-income populations in Ontario, Alberta, Nova Scotia, and British Columbia. Eligibility criteria for this study included (1) parents of children who had asthma and/or other respiratory health problems; and (2) low-income as determined using Statistics Canada's low-income cut-offs (Statistics Canada, 2015). The ethnic backgrounds of participants included Indigenous (First Nation, Métis), African, African-American, Asian (Filipino, Chinese), and Caucasian. Most parents (88 per cent) who participated in this intervention were mothers. Fifty-two per cent of parents were married, 32 per cent were single, and 16 per cent were divorced, separated, or widowed. English-language proficiency was "fluent" for 64 per cent of the parents and "good" for 36 per cent. Most parents indicated that their sole source of income was full-time work (48 per cent), followed by government assistance (24 per cent), other (16 per cent), and part-time work (12 per cent).

An eight-session (weekly or biweekly) support-education intervention was conducted over three months. The intervention was implemented online using a secure platform (GoToMeeting©). The sessions were facilitated by trained peer mentors and health professionals. Low-income families who did not have access to computers or the internet were given low-cost tablets and internet access. Most parents were not familiar with computers or the GoToMeeting© software. To facilitate participation, low-income parents were driven to a local community centre where they were guided by a peer mentor in using the online support program (e.g., logging in, connecting to the internet). This strategy increased participants' confidence. Once computer literate, parents were able to log in from their homes. A peer mentor was available by phone to enable parents to connect with the group and "troubleshoot" before each online support session. Parent participation in the eight online support-group sessions ranged from 73 to 89 per cent (average 79 per cent).

Group interviews and individual interviews, conducted with parents at post-test, yielded qualitative data on perceived impacts of the intervention, factors influencing its impacts, satisfaction with the intervention, and recommended changes. Individual in-depth interviews were conducted initially. Three group interviews subsequently reached parents who did not participate in individual interviews. Quantitative data on health-related outcomes were elicited by standardized measures administered individually, pre-intervention and post-intervention, via telephone to parents engaged in the online support-education program. Sixty-five per cent of parents completed both pre- and post-test measures.

Intervention Impacts

Decreased Isolation

Some low-income parents found it comforting to learn that others experienced similar challenges, as one parent stated: "Well it's been very helpful to see that I'm not alone, and that there are many people who are facing the same challenges that I'm facing, and to know that I'm not the only person going through some of the unique challenges."

Some parents previously felt isolated because they did not have anyone who could understand their demanding life situation. Parents noted that other low-income parents' stories about how they dealt with their children's medical conditions were helpful. Paired t-test analysis of pre- and post-intervention perceptions of social isolation or loneliness (as measured by the UCLA Loneliness Scale [D. Russell, 1996]) pointed to a decline in perceptions of loneliness following the support program (although not statistically significant).

Improved Coping

Parent participants reported gaining new information that helped them manage their children's health conditions. Some parents learned strategies to reduce stress when their children were sick. These low-income parents benefited from receiving accurate scientific knowledge from health professionals, including advice on how to administer medications. They learned ways of empowering children, seeking support, other coping strategies when monetary resources were low, and appropriate actions in emergencies. Parent participants said that their ability to cope with problems arising from their children's health condition increased after attending online support-group sessions. One parent explained: "I do feel better able to deal with my son's asthma. I was … connected with some great resources and some wonderful ladies."

Parents explained that they were able to plan better for expenses linked to caring for their children with respiratory problems. Participants learned how to seek help from spouses and others, such as their children's teacher and daycare staff. A mother shared: "Right now I know where to get help. I know where to run to if I had any emergency."

Parents maintained that their anxiety and stress was reduced by the intervention. Group members shared different perspectives regarding strategies to deal with physical, emotional, and mental challenges. Discussions about coping successes served as affirmational support.

Increased Knowledge

Parents reported that they learned from health professionals, because most had previous misconceptions regarding their children's respiratory problems. Knowledge gained from the support group also helped parents manage their own health. Participants learned from their peers and appreciated the opportunity to share their knowledge. One parent mentioned that their low-income environment was detrimental because she lived in subsidized housing and she had neighbours who smoked. Through support-group discussions, she learned how to effectively use her air filter. Another parent mentioned learning that her daughter's medication nebulizer mask should be changed at age six. Parents planned to implement the knowledge gained from these online group sessions in managing their children's health conditions, as one parent explained:

> Sometimes I feel like I don't have enough resources because it's very challenging having a child with asthma and allergies, but I have been given some great suggestions on how to utilize my very limited financial resources in the most effective way possible from some of the participants within the group, as well as some group leaders [who] have given some great suggestions too. I feel a lot more capable than I did previously.

Implications for Service Providers

This study also investigated service providers' perceptions of service and program inequities for low-income families with children facing chronic health conditions. Health and social service providers representing various disciplines/roles (e.g., asthma and cystic fibrosis clinic staff, family support workers, telehealth staff, pharmacists, community health workers, respiratory therapists, youth workers) and diverse service agencies (e.g., homeless programs, child services, churches, pediatric clinics) who work with people affected by both poverty and health problems were interviewed.

Enhanced Communication

Service providers' and policy influencers' suggestions for improved programs and policies focused on helping families cope with caring for a child with respiratory health problems, as well as barriers linked to low incomes. Service providers recommended that health professionals provide more information to low-income families about their children's conditions, management, and control. Some believed health professionals need improved communication skills to work with low-income families.

> Your style, manner, approach and the way you say things are unacceptable and inappropriate and you don't need to talk to people like they're stupid ... they're overwhelmed with all that's on their plate. They're not stupid just because they come here by bus or taxi or walk with their seven children. (Family support worker)

Policy influencers suggested heightening public awareness of barriers faced by low-income people affected by respiratory or other health conditions and increasing knowledge of provincial health benefit program providers, as one stated: "There's obviously a need for education, not only of parents but also of ... service providers ... because sometimes it is a lack of awareness." Service providers recommended relationship building in order to understand and meet the needs of low-income families. Strong relationships facilitate trust and communication between low-income families and service providers, and help tailor support to specific needs and capabilities of vulnerable parents.

Support to Access Resources

Service providers maintained that low-income parents and families need support to locate and access available resources. Complicated intake forms, language barriers, delays between referrals, lack of coordination among services, child care, and transportation posed barriers. They suggested that supports should be provided to low-income families following use of emergency health services. Policy influencers expressed particular concern for new immigrants and families just above low-income cut-offs who are isolated and less likely to be connected to services or supports.

> Where we need to get better ... is helping people navigate the system ... how can we better connect people ... here's how you access education, here's how you access this, here's what health link is for ... connecting

the dots for people because there are a lot of services that aren't being accessed. (Policy influencer)

Community Outreach

Some service providers and policy influencers recommended that child health services be linked to community programs for low-income families to improve accessibility and acceptability, and to alleviate language or cultural barriers, as one policy influencer pointed out: "Targeting the people that actually work with [low-income] people one on one ... Get it to the frontline staff (social workers, doctors) that work with them, get that information straight to them so they can tell the client faster and cut ... the bureaucracy out of it." Education-support for children in schools was recommended as an inclusive strategy to avoid isolating low-income children. Other suggested strategies included providing meals during health programs or childcare to help low-income parents who are forced to bring the siblings of the child with health problems to health services.

Proactive Support

Service providers suggested focusing on a few relevant points, once a relationship is built, to help low-income families who cannot otherwise access respiratory health education. A service provider recommended a change in perspective: "We have to get rid of ... wanting to tell them everything ... education would happen one little bit at a time."

Service providers asserted that resources should be allocated to supporting low-income families consistently, not solely during crises, to improve quality of life and reduce parent's health care expenses. Support services might cost more initially, but would be less expensive in the long term than frequent visits to the emergency room. In this context, service providers recommended proactive supports suitable for low-income families' needs and capabilities.

> They can't afford it because what they get for living is next to nothing. Do we then pay millions of dollars in health care later for these people who are sick, or do we help them now and reduce the severity of what they are sick with by putting in proper supports? Which is going to cost society least in the long run and be better for the person that you're working with? (Service provider)

Service providers and policy influencers recommended facilitating parent participation in health programs by providing transportation, time off work, and child care. Empowering low-income parents who feel marginalized, vulnerable and overwhelmed, to see value in sharing their experiences and their knowledge would help them adopt programs.

> Help them be aware of why it's important to include them … what kind of impact they're going to have on the policies and procedures, so instead of just talking to them about … services that they might need, it's also following up with them … because if they don't see that impact they're not going to continue. (Youth worker).

Service providers emphasized the importance of sharing insights based on low-income peoples' first-hand experiences, consulting with low-income communities, and including low-income people on advisory groups. A support worker for special needs children noted: "Lots of times I hear from families and I think 'Wow! Your thoughts and opinions are so profound, like you've got such good information. Would you be willing to participate in … to sit on … to share your story?'" Another service provider contended, "I think people have to be consulted from the grass-roots level."

Health service providers stated that they face obstacles to connecting low-income families with requisite resources and struggle to ensure comprehensive care. These professionals are impeded by a lack of coordination between diverse systems and sectors. They recognized the risks, vulnerabilities, and inequities in resources, yet when they encountered challenges to ensuring continuity of care for low-income families, they overcame the silo-nature of salient systems and promoted accessibility of resources. Service providers recommended minimizing language and cultural barriers to preventive supports; improving access to education; reducing environmental triggers; enhancing housing conditions; covering medication costs for children; following up after medical emergencies; and providing information about available supports.

The online intervention program presented in this chapter provided support and education to low-income parents with children who had respiratory health conditions. Parents reported improved coping skills and an increased knowledge of child health conditions and care strategies. Enhanced access to information about health conditions can reduce health inequities experienced by this high-risk group. Caregivers, peers, and teachers should be given knowledge and tools to help them empathize, understand, and assist these vulnerable parents in condition management. Parents who did not have social support reported higher levels of stress and anxiety. A recent report reveals that parents of chronically ill children experience more mental health problems than parents of unaffected children, and that these parents need focused interventions that mitigate harmful parent health outcomes (Cohn et al., 2020). As social support is a coping resource, parent participants in the online support intervention maintained that they coped better with adverse conditions linked to poverty and respiratory health problems.

Implications

This chapter demonstrated how a community model of care could promote social support and diminish parents' negative experiences with the health system which decrease accessibility. Indeed, improving community capacity enhances health equity (PHAC, 2008). Relevant strategies for reducing the complex burdens of chronic conditions require a comprehensive, coordinated public health approach that raises public awareness, increases capacity of community organizations, and encourages partnerships between vulnerable parents and health professionals. As families of children with health conditions are at heightened risk of economic adversity, due to increased pressures on family resources and diminished availability for employment, programs that address these demands require income supplementation and childcare assistance (Lukemeyer et al., 2004) to support parents' ability to provide care (Vonneilich et al., 2016). Poverty is multidimensional and dynamic and connected to social and economic exclusion, which emphasizes the importance of social support (Shimmin, 2020).

Programs, like our support intervention, can inform and educate affected parents, which can facilitate access to support and provide support opportunities to parents, and in turn have an enduring positive effect on physical and mental health (Vonneilich et al., 2016). This chapter provided insight into services needed, and information to guide development of support programs not only for low-income parents with chronically ill children but also other vulnerable groups.

9 Indigenous Parents and Caregivers Caring for Children with Chronic Health Conditions

MIRIAM J. STEWART AND
R. LISA BOURQUE BEARSKIN

Current trends point to significant increases in the population of Indigenous peoples in Canada, and to the corresponding need for improved health care services. Almost 5 per cent of the overall population self-identify as First Nations, Inuit, or Métis in Canada, with rapid growth at four times the rate of the non-Indigenous population (Statistics Canada, 2018b). Since 2006, there has been a 42.5 per cent increase in Indigenous peoples, with expected population growth to exceed 2.5 million within the next twenty years. This accelerated growth of the Indigenous population underscores expanding health inequalities (Pahwa et al., 2015). The state of Indigenous peoples' health serves as a powerful example of the social determinants of health (Canadian Nurses Association, 2014a).

Indigenous people are over-represented among the poor and disadvantaged. The average total income of men and women identified as "Aboriginal" in 2016 was 71 per cent of the average income of non-Indigenous men and 81 per cent of non-Indigenous women (Statistics Canada, 2019). Extreme poverty, low levels of education, low literacy rates, and poor housing limit Indigenous parents from building healthy lives for themselves and their children (UNICEF, 2009). While educational attainment is on the rise at high school and post-secondary levels, the Indigenous population still lags behind the non-Indigenous population (Statistics Canada, 2018b). Indigenous families live in diverse family configurations, including multigenerational homes, with 17.9 per cent of children living with grandparents (twice the rate of non-Indigenous children) and 34 per cent of children with a lone parent (compared with 17 per cent of non-Indigenous children). Indigenous families are also younger, larger, and include more extended family members compared to non-Indigenous families with children, which can be sources of strength as well as challenges in children's development (Halseth & Greenwood, 2019).

Unfortunately, many Indigenous people continue to face health risks alongside systemic discrimination in health care delivered to First Nations, Inuit, and Métis populations. The growing health inequities facing Indigenous peoples requires urgent action to address the legacy of disproportionate health burdens carried by Indigenous peoples. In Canada and elsewhere, Indigenous peoples are affected by major health problems at higher rates than non-Indigenous populations (National Collaboration Centre for Aboriginal Health [NCCAH], 2013). Indigenous Canadians have a significantly and consistently shorter life expectancy than the average non-Indigenous household population (Tjepkema et al., 2019) and experience higher rates of preventable chronic diseases compared with non-Indigenous Canadians (Gionet & Roshanafshar, 2015; King, 2010). Health challenges include high infant, child, and maternal morbidity and mortality; heavy infection disease burdens; social problems, illnesses, and deaths linked to the misuse of alcohol and other drugs; accidents, poisonings, interpersonal violence, homicides, and suicides; cigarette smoking; malnutrition; and diseases caused by environmental contamination. Although the basic causes of illness are similar for Indigenous and non-Indigenous peoples, the burden of disease, disability, and death is consistently greater for Indigenous people than it is for non-Indigenous people (Gracey & King, 2009).

Chapters 2, 3, and 6 explored physical and mental health issues facing Indigenous children. Asthma and allergies are particularly prevalent in the Indigenous population. Biological and sociological environmental factors influence the development and treatment of these conditions. Hospitalization and health care utilization rates are high while many do not receive necessary treatment, and ethnicity and discrimination are influencing factors (chapter 2). Chapter 3 highlighted health disparities linked to mental health issues and the prevalence of psychological distress among Indigenous children, and reviewed factors influencing mental health of Indigenous children (e.g., family environments, discrimination). Health issues linked to type 2 diabetes and sexually transmitted and blood-borne infections among Indigenous adolescents were introduced in chapter 6 along with examples of recent intervention programs.

In a review of studies from Canada, Australia, and New Zealand, it was found that parents' access to multidisciplinary health services for First Nations children with a chronic condition is critical for the children's health, but disparities and inequality in health systems have been virtually impossible to eliminate for First Nations people globally (Coombes et al., 2018). Indigenous parents of children with chronic health conditions, like asthma, could benefit from information about health risks and strategies to help their children manage risks and from access to relevant support. Moreover, increasing Indigenous parents' involvement in planning, decision-making, design, and implementation of programs, services, and financial resources could help parents meet their needs (Institute of Fiscal Studies and Democracy [IFSD], 2020; Reading & Wien, 2009). In 2017, the Canadian Government asked how the First Nations Child and Family Service program could be reformed. Most respondents reported that families could be healthier and happier with more culturally sensitive services for Indigenous parents and children (Indigenous Services Canada, 2018).

The aim of this chapter is to report on our studies, which bridged research gaps by examining health and health care inequities from the perspective of parents of Indigenous children and adolescents with respiratory and allergic conditions. This research will reveal that inadequate social support, social exclusion and isolation, income gaps, institutional barriers, and policy limitations influence the health behaviours of Indigenous children and their parents, as well as their use of health services. This chapter will also describe culturally appropriate and accessible support-education programs designed and delivered by Indigenous peers and health professionals based on the needs and preferences of Indigenous parents.

Culturally Responsive Approaches

The first study (M. Stewart, Castleden et al., 2015) was conducted by an interdisciplinary research team encompassing Indigenous researchers and knowledge users, and employed a multimethod participatory research design (Bergold & Thomas, 2012), with guidance from Indigenous community advisory committees. Consistent with principles of participatory research (Bergold & Thomas, 2012; Boffa et al., 2011), parents of Indigenous children specified their preferred type, format, and substantive content of support interventions; helped select specific interventions; and suggested changes for future interventions. The Indigenous community advisory committees in each of the three study sites (Alberta, Manitoba, Nova Scotia) guided selection, screening, and training of project staff; amendment of interview guides and measures; identification of culturally appropriate recruitment strategies; design of the intervention; identification of optimum intervention outcomes; and relevant knowledge translation strategies. The community advisory committee in Alberta, comprised of ten Indigenous community leaders, provided guidance on the development, implementation, and evaluation of the study. In Manitoba, the research team formalized a partnership with Dakota Tipi First Nation. The Elders determined that this community-based participatory project, with previously secured support from the Assembly of Manitoba Chiefs and its research ethics supervisors, was consistent with the community's health goals. Relationships were also developed with five Mi'kmaq communities in Nova Scotia, through each community's health director. Ethics approval was confirmed from the Mi'kmaw Ethics Watch, an independent process to ensure that research involving Mi'kmaq people is culturally appropriate and safeguards Indigenous knowledge (Mi'kmaw Ethics Watch, 1999).

Indigenous Parent Support Needs and Intervention Preferences

Collectively, seventy-seven parents of Indigenous children with asthma agreed to participate in individual interviews to identify preferences regarding support interventions (Alberta, $n = 51$; Manitoba, $n = 9$; Nova Scotia, $n = 17$). The adults, primarily women, were parents or guardians of Indigenous children diagnosed with chronic respiratory conditions. In three cases, participating parents had Indigenous children through second marriages or adoption. In Alberta, fifteen parents from three Métis communities (Buffalo Lake, Kikano, and Elizabeth), thirty-three parents from nine First Nations communities (Blood Tribe, Cold Lake First Nation, Enoch Cree Nation, Fort McKay, Kehewin, Whitefish Lake First Nation, Siksika Nation, Samson Cree Nation, and Tsuu T'ina Nation), and three Caucasian parents of Indigenous children in Alberta participated in these interviews.

Trained Indigenous interviewers conducted in-depth individual interviews with parents. Moreover, twenty-five parents (twelve selected from individual interview participants and thirteen additional First Nations and Métis parents) participated in two follow-up group interviews, one in an urban site and one in a rural setting. A semi-structured interview guide was developed to elicit parents' perspectives, challenges, barriers, and support needs. During group interviews, participants received a synopsis of results from individual interviews and were asked if the interpretations were accurate and appropriate. In Manitoba, nine caregivers participated in a group interview. Seven of these caregivers self-identified as Dakota, one was Métis, and one was a Euro-Canadian parent of an Indigenous child. In the east, Mi'kmaq families were recruited from across five Nova Scotia communities (Eskasoni, Waycobah, Wagmatcook, Potlotek, and Membertou in Unama'ki, Cape Breton). Interviews were conducted in English with occasional, spontaneous use of Mi'kmaq. A semi-structured individual interview guide elicited parents' perceptions of (a) their caregiving demands and challenges requiring support; (b) their coping strategies, including support seeking; (c) their support needs and support resources; (d) programs serving parents of Indigenous children/adolescents; (e) gaps in available supports and services; (f) preferences for culturally congruent support interventions and; (g) culturally appropriate intervention outcomes. Group interviews with parents/guardians were conducted subsequently to verify and clarify specific features of recommended support interventions.

Overall findings from our assessment study indicated that these parents lacked information and financial support to manage their children's health conditions. They were concerned about mould in their homes and environmental risks. Dusty roads, insufficient federal support of housing, overcrowded multigenerational housing, proximal air-polluting industry, poverty, and concomitant risky health behaviours were identified as contributors to poor respiratory health. Parents relied on both lived experience and medical advice when managing their child's health condition, and reported insufficient community-level knowledge and resources. They identified geographic distance as a major barrier to accessing supports outside their communities. Moreover, support resources external to their communities were available only in English and were often not covered by the Non-Insured Health Benefits Program.

Family gatherings and cultural celebrations and ceremonies are important in Indigenous culture. However, First Nations parents reported barriers to participation in some events because tobacco smoke, pets, animal hides, and fur (present at many traditional Indigenous gatherings) are common triggers for asthma attacks and allergic reactions. Parents expressed concern about illness exacerbations linked to exposure to allergens related to cultural practices (e.g., smudging ceremony, incense), and the environment (e.g., air pollution, dust, mould, ground fires). Mould caused by spring flooding, poor housing design and construction, and inadequate drainage was common. While not the norm, one parent's strategy for managing environmental risks was described by an adolescent with asthma: "My dad got these guys to check my house, and I don't know what was wrong with it but I think there was, like, mould and lots of dust. So he got it renovated and I've been pretty good since then."

Many young Indigenous mothers blamed themselves for their children's conditions. Moreover, some family members as well as health and social service professionals attributed these respiratory problems to poor parenting practices and smoking. One mother said, "How many times a social service was called on me because I'm an Aboriginal woman, you know, to come to make sure I wasn't smoking in my house" (First Nations mother of adolescents with asthma and allergies).

Some parents lacked support outside their family and indicated that community access to information about these health conditions contributed to their support deficits. The perceived stigma of chronic illness compounded parents' sense of isolation and exclusion. Additionally, many parents believed that the stigma of being Indigenous impeded access to needed services and supports. They wanted support from peers who understood their problems and could help them cope: "I could deal with the medical stuff fine but I really needed family or somebody to talk to. I really needed to cry to somebody and say, 'I'm scared about my baby'" (First Nations parent of child with asthma and allergies).

Most parents experienced gaps in information. Inadequate information about use of prescribed medication was evident. Parents did not understand the terminology used by health professionals to describe their children's health conditions and lacked information about short- and long-term effects of inflammation on lungs, causes of asthma, and triggers for allergic reactions. These Indigenous parents seemed to have low self-efficacy and believed that their skills for dealing with their children's chronic conditions were inadequate.

Some parents indicated that health-related problems such as school absenteeism, fatigue, hyperactivity, and concentration challenges were attributed by teachers and health professionals to Indigenous culture rather than the medical condition of treatment. Many parents complained that education and support were not culturally appropriate. They sought emotional and practical support from Elders. However, culturally congruent support was not available through health-care encounters or education. Parents were aware that smoking aggravated asthma and that asthma abated when they stopped smoking or smoked outdoors. However, some found it difficult to ask friends and relatives to smoke outdoors: "We used to smoke in the house and she would get a runny nose and ear infections a lot, so we stopped smoking in the house and she doesn't have so many ear infections and runny nose" (First Nations parent of adolescent with allergies and asthma).

Lack of transportation imposed major obstacles. In many rural communities, distance from hospitals and delays in ambulance service were significant barriers. Medical transportation provided in First Nations communities requires pre-booking and is often unavailable on short notice. Additionally, many single mothers experienced significant conflict between their busy work schedules and the time required to manage their children's health care appointments, as these young parents did not have reliable transportation, childcare, home telephones, or cell phones. Parents juggled jobs and responsibilities at home, leaving little time for trips to specialist appointments in distant cities. Children's school and extra-curricular activities also precluded parents' participation in parental health education and support programs.

Several parents expressed concern about underdiagnosis, reporting that asthma was incorrectly diagnosed as bronchitis or a short-term acute condition. Although these Indigenous parents described significant symptoms, only those who lived in the city or were well educated were referred to a specialist for testing. Parents received conflicting advice from different health professionals. Some used traditional healing methods and others were curious about how traditional medicines would interact with physician-prescribed medications. Several parents described discriminatory, non-supportive encounters with health care providers because they were Indigenous: "He still has to use that machine, a Ventolin machine … We knew he was allergic to cats and dogs, because when he was around them he reacted, but he's never been tested … They [the doctors] weren't very helpful" (Métis parent of adolescents with asthma and allergies).

Parents who did not have access to pharmaceutical insurance found it difficult to pay for prescribed medications. Some parents reported that physicians recommended emergency room visits if they needed access to medications. "He's had it since he was a baby. He was diagnosed pretty early. It was very stressful because he was in the hospital a lot … I didn't have a job that had coverage, so his medication was pretty expensive" (Métis parent of adolescents with asthma and allergies – rural).

Parents believed that medication policy for Indigenous people should be less complex. Some young parents discovered that their child did not have First Nations medication coverage because government forms had not been signed or their child's treaty status was being contested:

> I basically go months without health coverage for them, and it's a struggle, because they get sick and I don't know where to take them and where to get their medicine. I have to pay [for] their medicine, and that's so hard to do when you're struggling to find money for it. (First Nations mother of two children with asthma and allergies)

Parents wanted support to understand and manage respiratory health problems; information on use of prescribed, over-the-counter, and traditional medications; advice regarding communication strategies with health professionals; and insights from other Indigenous parents on the management of their children's health conditions. They required advice from health professionals in the system, along with support from both Indigenous peers and Indigenous professionals. Parents desired increased information and educational resources to help manage their children's conditions. Parents contended that they needed culturally appropriate support, education, and childcare during support- intervention sessions. Recommended support interventions included education and support groups.

Culturally Congruent Support Interventions

Forty parents/caregivers of Indigenous children with asthma and allergies participated in the pilot support interventions (Alberta, $n = 20$; Nova Scotia, $n = 17$; Manitoba, $n = 3$). All the interventions were designed to provide support and education (M. Stewart, Castleden et al., 2015). Specific interventions for each site were determined by Indigenous parent preferences expressed in assessment interviews regarding intervention mode; supporters; timing, frequency, and duration; and discussion topics. All support programs were co-facilitated by trained Indigenous peer mentors, Indigenous health professionals, or Indigenous Elders. To accommodate the preferences of parents in different communities, diverse support interventions were designed, implemented, and pilot tested in different provinces. To enhance accessibility of these interventions regardless of socio-economic status and geographic location, transportation and childcare were provided when needed.

In Alberta, eight Indigenous parents/caregivers from one rural First Nations community and twelve from an urban centre, primarily First Nations and Métis, participated in support interventions. Consistent with the preferences of these parents, face-to-face support-group interventions, supplemented by Telehealth, were implemented and tested. Eight support-group sessions were delivered through Telehealth to rural Indigenous parents. To accommodate distance, oneHealth (a Telehealth portal sponsored by First Nations and Inuit Health) was used to link rural and remote First Nations communities to health professionals who had expertise relevant to their children's health conditions. Parents met at the health centre to interact with health experts and peers on Telehealth. Topics included keeping homes free of allergens and mould, avoiding asthma triggers, culturally relevant and safe use of traditional medicine, and tobacco, among others. After each formal Telehealth session ended, parents at the rural health centre discussed implications for the management of their child's condition with a trained Indigenous peer mentor and health professional. The intervention exerted impacts beyond participants. As sessions were available to all First Nations and Métis health centres through the oneHealth portal, thirty Indigenous people (on average) at fifteen rural health centres also participated in each session.

For those twelve parents in the Alberta urban centre, eight face-to-face support-group sessions were delivered by a trained Indigenous peer mentor and health professional weekly at an inner-city school with an infused Indigenous curriculum. These parents discussed topics similar to those requested by the eight rural parents, but they also wanted information on urban services and supports. Three parents from the Dakota Tipi tribe in Manitoba attended face-to-face support-group sessions. In Nova Scotia, seventeen Mi'kmaq rural parents participated in a two-day asthma camp with their children, which included Indigenous ceremonies (smudging, prayer); cultural activities (drum making, drumming, singing, dancing); entertainment (games, art, relay races, movie night); social support (informal networking opportunities); and education (asthma awareness training, expert guest speakers).

To test the impacts of these support programs, data collection strategies included standardized quantitative measures, individual qualitative interviews, a sharing circle, and a group interview. Similar post-intervention interview guides were used across all three provincial sites. All parents were interviewed individually prior to and following these support interventions. A ten-item semi-structured interview guide elicited qualitative data regarding intervention processes, perceived intervention impacts, and recommended changes. Three standardized quantitative measures were also administered to parents to test the impacts of the intervention: the UCLA Loneliness Scale (D. Russell, 1996), the Personal Resource Questionnaire (Weinert, 2003), and the Proactive Coping Inventory (Greenglass et al., 1999). These were deemed culturally appropriate by the Indigenous advisers and had good psychometric properties. These quantitative pre-test and post-test measures were administered only at the Alberta site, consistent with Indigenous community advisory committees' preferences, whereas qualitative interview guides were used across provinces.

In Alberta, urban Indigenous parents reported significantly more social support resources than rural participants at pre-test. Loneliness scores were significantly lower at post-test following the support intervention than at pre-test. Social support scores increased for both rural and urban participants after the support interventions. An Indigenous mother explained how the program fostered social support between peers:

> [The support program] helps because ... some people are terrified and they don't want to talk about it [problems] in a public setting but when you're [in support program] ... you ... say, "Hey, it's okay." Then you [can] direct them to who would know the answers that they're looking for.

Support-seeking coping also increased post-intervention (not statistically significant). In post-test qualitative interviews (that extended and refined the data elicited by the quantitative measures), parents reported that they were more prepared to seek support following the intervention, but that support resources were only minimally available in their communities. Indigenous parents described the need for community health centres to be champions.

Rural parents in Alberta appreciated meeting on Telehealth, although oneHealth was available only from 9 a.m. to 5 p.m. In post-intervention interviews, urban parents contended that their experience with peer support from the support-group intervention was so positive that they wanted similar support resources relevant to other challenges in their lives. Participants reported that they learned from the inquiries of other parents in support groups, as a mother explained: "People ask questions that you don't even think about asking and then they'll say, 'Oh yeah that, you know, that's another thing that I should have asked and your questions are being answered.'"

The delivery of health information within the context of traditional cultural practices and lifestyles was appreciated. Indigenous parents also valued the positive "demystification" of research by the support intervention activities. According to parents in Nova Scotia, the camp reduced their loneliness; improved asthma support and education; enabled social learning; enhanced friendships and family communication; and taught strategies for communicating with other community members. Participants suggested that future community-based health interventions could be undertaken in the language used by their Indigenous community.

Accessible, Culturally Appropriate Support-Education Programs

Despite efforts by the health care sector to deliver culturally responsive and appropriate health knowledge to Indigenous populations, the experience of individual and systemic discrimination when seeking care is prominent (Allan & Smylie 2015; Goodman et al., 2017; Government of British Columbia, 2020; Phillips-Beck et al. 2020). In response to this growing concern, Indigenous nursing leadership in Canada recognizes that Indigenous knowledge and understanding is needed and health care providers' approach to delivering services to Indigenous families in Canada must be improved. These advancements must be informed by both socio-historical contexts and unique complexities of policy and health care funding (Aboriginal Nurses Association of Canada, 2014;

Bourque Bearskin et al., 2021; Canadian Nurses Association, 2014b; Du
Paula & Rabbitskin, 2018). Nurses and other health professionals are
called on to reflect on their "colonial" worldview and its influence on
their interpretation and delivery of services. If nurses deny the legiti-
macy of Indigenous history in Canada, they subsequently deny Indigenous peoples' capacity and human rights to ethical health care services
(Bourque Bearskin et al., 2020).

Although leaders in many health organizations have committed
to working towards equity and reconciliation in health care, which
includes a focus on cultural safety and the incorporation of traditional
medicine and healing practices, this vision is not yet fully realized (Redvers et al., 2019). Of growing significance are community calls for integration of traditional healing approaches within the current health
care model. Indigenous nursing leaders are assessing approaches to
developing policies and are changing practice in partnership with
Indigenous peoples to incorporate traditional healing, spiritual, and
cultural practices into health care (Caxaj et al., 2018; Marsh et al.,
2018; Sickle et al., 2003). A holistic, unified approach can contribute
to overcoming barriers and challenges facing Indigenous communities, consistent with Indigenous perspectives (NCCAH, 2017). Health
professionals should offer Indigenous children and their parents
time and space to respect their cultural beliefs regarding care options
(Towle et al., 2006). Public health efforts aimed at attending to health
conditions challenging Indigenous populations must consider the
unique contexts in which Indigenous people live (NCCAH, 2012). In
public health and clinical services, strategies to address social determinants of Indigenous child and parent health must recognize the social
circumstances and the restrictions that such circumstances place on
health (Browne et al., 2016).

Acknowledging differences in socio-economic circumstances and
lived world experiences of First Nations, Inuit, and Métis peoples, and
between status and non-status, on-reserve and off-reserve, as well as
urban and rural Indigenous populations is important (NCCAH, 2013).
Culturally appropriate and accessible support-education programs
delivered by Indigenous peers and health professionals are needed to
help reduce inequities and health service barriers. Information about
health conditions and condition management requires a cross-disciplinary
approach. Indigenous children and parents need to understand the
terminology used by health professionals to describe their children's
health conditions. Considering that Indigenous nations are grounded
in oral teachings, knowledge mobilization strategies such as infographics (images, charts, and minimal text providing clear topic overviews)

tend to be more effective in translating medical information. Other strategies include:

• Listen to the expressed immediate concerns of the family unit.
• Ask questions to better understand traditional healing and the use of traditional medicines.
• Ensure an environment of cultural humility and security that enables Indigenous parents to seek information free of judgments regarding identity, parenting skills, or living conditions.
• Support clients by booking transportation for health care appointments and referrals to non-insured health benefit plans.
• Teach clients how to ask questions so they understand the causes of their conditions, the strategies to manage treatment options, the use of medications, how to monitor side effects, and how to access emergency services.

Indigenous engagement in health policy design, planning, and delivery can yield more culturally responsive and accessible health care services, which in the long term will positively impact health outcomes (Lavoie et al., 2012). Wise practices incorporating Indigenous approaches revealed in this study highlight important features of care aimed at individual, systemic, and political (proximal, intermediate, and distal) determinants of health (Reading & Wein, 2009). Beginning with the individual level, both Indigenous clients and health practitioners should engage in authentic self-awareness while creating a shared vision for care plans; knowledge translation easily understood by the parents, the children, and the public; and advocacy for organizational change. Respectful, reciprocal, relevant, and responsible relationships that are grounded in a strengths-focused, rights-based, and non-hierarchical approach are important. Promotion of equity is central to decolonizing health care approaches (Bourque Bearskin et al., 2020; Kelly, 2011; Kenny, 2012; Kurtz, 2014; Reading & Wien, 2009).

Insufficient community level supports, inadequate educational resources, environmental vulnerability, and condition management barriers can be targeted through training for health professionals and culturally appropriate support-education programs delivered by Indigenous peoples. Health professionals are not typically trained to understand the perspectives of Indigenous peoples or to provide culturally appropriate care (Larson et al., 2011; L. Stewart & Nielsen, 2011). Some strategies aimed at enhancing culturally specific support-education include:

- Considering language, culture, and health together: "recognize the value of Aboriginal healing practices and use them in the treatment of Aboriginal patients ..." (Call to Action #22, Truth and Reconciliation Commission of Canada, 2015, p. 2).
- Alleviating environmental hazards such as dust, dirt roads, moulds, water, and air contamination.
- Eliminating barriers to health condition management such as access to hospital and emergency care; service delays through protracted referral processes; and limited financial resources for medications and equipment.

One effective way to address social-cultural pressures and lack of community knowledge and support for affected parents is to train Indigenous community health champions to develop culturally appropriate activities specific to their location. This helps reduce stigma, isolation, and social pressures.

Research Insights and Implications for Future Services

Grant funding from the Canadian Institutes of Health Research and from the Aboriginal Capacity and Developmental Research Environments for Aboriginal health research were significant contributors to the success of these studies. The multidisciplinary research team included researchers and collaborators from medicine, nursing, geography, law, and anthropology. Partnerships with First Nations and Métis communities and leaders, health professionals, researchers, and not-for-profit community organizations formed the foundations of these programs.

The support interventions explored in this chapter and in chapter 2 focused on Indigenous children have the potential to (1) improve relevance and uptake of health programs through support provisions informed by the needs and wishes of affected Indigenous children and parents; (2) enhance efficacy of health interventions by supplementing professional knowledge with credible experiential knowledge of peers; (3) expand the capacity of Indigenous children/adolescents and their parents to manage health problems and to support others; and (4) promote the use of accessible technologies for supporting Indigenous communities in addressing cultural and geographic inequities. As there is inadequate evidence on the effectiveness of different types of support interventions for Indigenous parents, and as participatory principles are vital in research engaging Indigenous people (Tri-Council, 2010), in our studies we invited Indigenous participants to select preferred interventions for specific settings (rural/urban). This important input resulted in the creation of culturally accessible support interventions that fostered resilience and coping strategies and transcended physical and geographic barriers. Parents of Indigenous children described enhanced support and reduced education needs following the interventions shared in this chapter. These perceived impacts are important given reports that social support gaps and poverty create significant disparities in life chances between Indigenous and non-Indigenous children, parents, and their families (Canadian Council of Child and Youth Advocates, 2011; NCCAH, 2017; Standing Senate Committee on Human Rights, 2007). First Nations, Inuit, and Métis populations, whether urban, rural, or remote, face many challenges in health, as health services frequently neglect to address health and social inequities (Browne et al., 2016).

Across our studies, Indigenous parents reported challenges with knowledge gaps, poverty, blame imposed on them for their children's illnesses, underdiagnosis, uncoordinated health care, disrespectful treatment, environmental problems, and lack of culturally appropriate support. Health care inequalities underlying societal and systemic barriers diminished support from traditional family and community sources. Poverty, limited health literacy, unemployment, negative encounters with health and social-service systems, discriminatory and racist attitudes of professionals, and cultural misunderstanding are barriers to timely and appropriate services (NCCAH, 2017; Postl et al., 2010; Phillips-Beck et al., 2020; Van Herk et al., 2011). Peer support interventions can improve the relevance, efficacy, and uptake of health programs by supplementing professional knowledge with the credible experiential knowledge of peers; enhancing the capacity of Indigenous parents to manage health challenges; and increasing accessibility to interventions that address cultural and geographic inequities. This "different strokes for different folks" strategy reflects participatory principles and seems more acceptable and accessible than a generic "one size fits all" approach to interventions for vulnerable parents of Indigenous children.

Although organizations are moving towards more cultural responsiveness to meet the needs of Indigenous populations, there is still a long way to go. A systemic shift is required to dismantle structural inequities and ensure that parents and families with Indigenous children needing health services for chronic conditions are treated respectfully (Richmond & Cook, 2016). Service providers can enhance the delivery of culturally competent care if they understand the diversity and cultural backgrounds of Indigenous parents and children (Coombes et al., 2018). Indigenous health practitioners face distinctive challenges associated with accessing and applying both Indigenous and Western knowledge and evidence in their practice (Rogers et al., 2019). The development of

Indigenous-led programs offer strengths-based and proactive approaches to support families and provide opportunities to become successful parents (Wright et al., 2019). Indigenous peoples' involvement is essential in the creation of family support services that address Indigenous social determinants within a primary health care model. Aboriginal parents must have access to supportive services, resources, and preventive programming to authentically address unique systemic and structural forces that have negatively impacted their lives (Halseth & Murdock, 2020; Reading & Wien, 2009).

10 Innovative Programs for Parents Coping with Health Inequities Informed by Research Insights

NICOLE LETOURNEAU AND MIRIAM J. STEWART

Our studies, conducted in large programs of research spanning numerous provinces, revealed an abundance of evidence about the detrimental impacts of health and social problems on vulnerable children/adolescents and their parents. For both parents and their children, negative impacts included loneliness, social isolation, and support deficiencies. In what follows, insights are shared from studies conducted with diverse vulnerable groups facing health and social disadvantages, including refugee new parents (Makwarimba et al., 2013; M. Stewart, Makwarimba et al., 2015), parents affected by post-partum depression (Letourneau et al., 2015, 2012, 2007), mothers who suffered from partner violence (Letourneau et al., 2011), and parents of children with respiratory problems (M. Stewart, Castleden et al., 2015). The aim of this chapter is to present the knowledge mobilization strategies used in our research to (1) engage these vulnerable populations of knowledge users directly affected by health inequities and health problems in informing the development and adaptation of accessible relevant support-education interventions; (2) enable decision-makers (i.e., program planners, policy influencers, service providers/managers) to inform the design, testing, and transfer of support-education interventions; and (3) identify the implications of support-education interventions for programs, policies, and practice in health and health-related sectors.

Early Knowledge Translation by Engaging Knowledge Users

The studies described in this chapter employ integrated knowledge translation methods (Straus et al., 2013) to involve stakeholders in refinement of research questions, validation of research results, engagement in intervention program development, and end-of-study dissemination. Throughout our support intervention research, knowledge users and decision-makers in varied health and health-related sectors were engaged in discussions of outreach, communication, and recruitment strategies pertinent to health challenges of vulnerable populations. Key agencies and organizations were consulted (consistent with principles of integrated knowledge translation) and knowledge was exchanged with them during the early phases of research. Stakeholders, such as knowledge users, participant representatives, and decision-makers shared their perspectives, expertise, knowledge, concerns, and questions to inform development of relevant research programs, which reflect participatory research principles. These early interactions encouraged researchers to check their assumptions about community and to consider the clinical relevance of their research questions, resulting in the refinement of studies to suit the community stakeholders' reported needs.

To illustrate, during the development of intervention studies focused on supporting Sudanese and Zimbabwean new parents (M. Stewart, Makwarimba et al., 2015), content of the interventions emerged from knowledge gaps identified by individual groups of refugee parents and reflected their unique ethnocultural support needs and intervention preferences. A Zimbabwean female mentor articulated the preferences expressed by many refugee new parents:

> They wanted to share challenges that they are facing; they wanted to find out how other participants deal with such challenges and what's the best way to deal with it like coping strategies; and some of them just wanted to find out where they can get more information in relation to their everyday challenges that they are facing.

Further, English-language barriers and health illiteracy issues surfaced and were met with the recommendation to provide translators for participants, and to offer translations of materials in the participants' first languages. This participatory approach ensured that refugee parent participants received information that filled their knowledge gaps, and enabled them to optimize their use of formal support services and their navigation of health, education, housing, financial, and other service systems. Sharing information and knowledge of available services enhanced their sense of empowerment and confidence to function in Canadian society.

Similarly, we engaged with mothers affected by postpartum depression in developing Mothers Offering Mentorship and Support (MOMS) Link, a telephone-based support-education program designed to reduce depressive symptoms (Letourneau et al., 2007). One mother described how she could benefit from such peer support: "Another woman that had been through it: that's the kind of support I was looking for. What I really didn't want was for my mom or my husband to carry it all, because I would worry as much about that."

We also interviewed fathers, whose partners were affected by postpartum depression, to identify their perceived support-education needs (Letourneau et al., 2012). Fathers confirmed that they could also benefit from peer support. As one said: "It's like this big pressure. This massive amount of weight of things, thoughts, and feelings and just by expressing them to another human being, it was like giving a lot of it away ... I don't know, it's a weird analogy I guess. It's like here, take this [burden]."

Furthermore, engagement with stakeholders enabled the identification of key informants for intervention development and participants for intervention program testing. These stakeholders not only possessed expert knowledge of the sources of potential participants but also ensured that the interventions were designed to support parents deemed most in need. Stakeholders' embeddedness in the early phases of research, as part of the research team, promoted a sense of study ownership and commitment to the study's success.

Another example emerged from our study of the support-education needs experienced by mothers affected by intimate partner violence (Letourneau et al., 2011). In this study, we interviewed mothers affected by violence as well as their service providers. Service providers were drawn from diverse organizations, including transition and second-stage housing; victim services; counseling services; legal education services; legal aid; family and community resource centres; and provincial public health, mental health, and social services agencies. In addition to recognizing the need for support that promotes women's sense of dignity, service providers noted that affected mothers wanted support to "allow women to, or teach women again, how to nurture and truly bond with their children ... parenting techniques, whether you're in an abusive relationship or not, are a really valuable tool." Communications with stakeholders in service provision agencies fostered a sense of connection to the study, and ultimately contributed to successful end-of-study knowledge translation.

Knowledge Translation in Intervention Research Processes

Knowledge translation and exchange were essential strategies during our support intervention studies. Data were collected from participants and stakeholders to examine the intervention processes underpinning impacts identified through both quantitative and qualitative methods. Several studies serve as examples. Our study (M. Stewart, Castleden et al., 2015) focused on supporting Indigenous parents of children and adolescents with respiratory problems, highlighted the importance of sharing and receiving knowledge. Indigenous parents, many of whom had previous misconceptions regarding their children's health conditions, reported that they learned from health professionals in our support interventions, and that they benefited from the accurate scientific knowledge provided by health professional mentors. Participants also learned from support group peers, and shared perceived deficits in their knowledge of their children's health. Parents planned to implement the knowledge they gained from peer-support-group sessions in managing their own and their children's health conditions.

In our support intervention study with refugees from Sudan and Somalia, adult participants, many of whom were parents, preferred a combination of individual-level support for sharing personal information about sensitive issues and peer group support for exchanging information and discussing common problems facing refugees (Makwarimba et al., 2013). Another support intervention designed for low-income parents of children and adolescents with asthma revealed preferences for parent peer-support groups facilitated by knowledgeable professionals to provide information and emotional and affirmation support; to offer guidance; to interpret available information; and to translate this information into knowledge relevant to their situation (M. Stewart, Letourneau et al., 2011). A low-income parent explained the knowledge they gained:

> Sometimes I feel like I don't have enough resources because it's very challenging having a child with asthma and allergies, but I have been given some great suggestions on how to utilize my very limited financial resources in the most effective way possible from some of the participants within the group, as well ... some group leaders have given [me] some great suggestions too. I feel a lot more capable than I did previously.

In addition, vulnerable parents reported wanting support to advocate for improved programs and policies.

The Attachment and Child Health (ATTACH™) program emerged from our research on mothers' support-education needs when affected by intimate partner violence. Situated in a context of social support that ensured participant dignity, the program focused on helping mothers improve their ability to think about their children's feelings as essential precursors to healthy parent-child relationships, secure mother-child attachment, and optimal child development. Quantitative findings demonstrated program effectiveness (Letourneau et al., 2020), however, qualitative quotes from mothers and stakeholders from community agencies were most compelling in demonstrating intervention processes.

A mother who participated in the program commented: "It's working to help me think and teach my kids how others feel and think. It's helping with peers at school with my son. It also helped me work through issues with my son's dad." Another parent said: "In some situations when I'm upset, it made me think, why am I upset? Why is she [child] upset? I need to see from her eyes and just understand from her eyes, just to, you know, to communicate." Clearly, parents benefited from the process of direct knowledge exchange by being recognized and respected participants in the studies.

Innovative Knowledge Translation at End-of-Study

End-of-study methods for knowledge translation employed innovative methods for knowledge sharing that maximized stakeholder engagement and knowledge uptake. Following the completion of intervention studies, knowledge translation and mobilization is vital. Thus, the communication of research insights regarding support-education needs and preferences, and support intervention impacts and processes, was a key strategy in our studies. Familiar academic routes for sharing study insights were undertaken, including peer-reviewed journal publications, book chapters, textbooks, conference presentations, and fact sheets (Tsui et al., 2006). Subscribing to the adage that a picture is worth a thousand words, both fact sheets and presentations with stakeholders employed data visualization strategies, such as simplified graphics and figures that illustrated key concepts. Knowledge mobilization and translation strategies focused on sharing information with:

- Stakeholders who provide services for vulnerable populations;
- Policymakers who promote program development or make informed decisions based on research results; and
- Participants and other vulnerable populations who could share results with people in similar situations and be empowered to access salient support programs.

These knowledge translation activities were reciprocal as stakeholders, decision-makers, and knowledge users could suggest improvements for support services, implementation of similar programs, and future research and program directions. For example, we conducted a knowledge mobilization symposium with service providers for low-income families, policy influencers, decision-makers, and partner organizations to solicit input on sustainable, innovative, and accessible support-education programs for low-income children/adolescents with respiratory problems and their parents. Knowledge users across Canada from national, provincial, and municipal entities participated. In preparation for the symposium, appealing fact sheets summarizing key findings were shared, as well as more detailed reports. During the sessions, findings were presented and participants were invited to suggest dissemination targets, formats, and follow-up activities that would enhance impact.

We offered a similar conference following the initial research on mothers' support-education needs for managing postpartum depression (Letourneau et al., 2007). Indeed, the conference was a direct consequence of mothers' confirmation of the essential need for public awareness about postpartum depression:

> I think people in general need to be more aware. Some people may not even see it until their partner or their friend or their sister says, "You're not yourself." Other people around need to know, "Okay this is a possibility and these are the things you look for and this is what you can do."

In this spirit, the conference not only focused on drawing an audience that included policy decision-makers from the government and service providers from across Canada, but also emphasized learning for new mothers facing, or who had recently faced, postpartum depression.

Integrated knowledge translation strategies during and at the end-of-study must be multifaceted for maximum reach. Traditional peer-reviewed publications are essential. Meetings, such as symposia or conferences, foster face-to-face knowledge exchange at various stages in the research process, but may be most effective at end-of-study. Increasingly, social media is an avenue for knowledge exchange and dissemination used by researchers (Gruzd et al., 2012). Social media may be employed at every stage of the study, but its greatest value may be at the end when assessment insights and intervention impacts are accessible. Early on, stakeholders and participants may be updated regularly about study processes, including challenges and successes, and opportunities offered for bidirectional exchange on platforms such as Twitter (Choo et al., 2015), Facebook, or private sharing sites such as Slack (Keller et al., 2014). However, at end-of-study, social media may be most useful for sharing findings in novel ways with new audiences. Links to publications in peer-reviewed journals, as well as quick facts, infographics, or research highlights, can be posted to these social media sharing sites in order to relay findings to stakeholders, participants, and the wider community. Indeed, this approach may foster public discourse on research findings (Keller et al., 2014) and extend impacts. Findings may be shared and reshared, reaching far more stakeholders and knowledge users than traditional methods allow.

This approach has been undertaken with great success in our parent-focused ATTACH™ and MOMS Link studies. For example, opinion editorials summarizing findings from MOMS Link and information relevant to postpartum depression were prepared and shared with media outlets across Canada. One such opinion editorial was published in Canada's national newspaper, the *Globe and Mail*, and featured on its online home page on 6 March 2017. It was the *Globe and Mail*'s most tweeted article that week and made the category of "Popular This Week," being shared more than 80 times, receiving more than 140 likes and comments, and reaching more than 13,000 people. Other opinion editorials have been published and republished online (e.g., HuffPost) and in traditional print media (e.g., the *Winnipeg Free Press*, *Hill Times*), typically placing in the top six Canadian news sources and reaching varied audiences from across Canada. Findings from the ATTACH™ study were summarized and shared in an interview available on the *Brain Child* podcast series on iTunes. The link to the series was tweeted out to the principal investigator's more than 20,000 Twitter followers, with many retweets, multiplying potential exposure to the study's findings.

Knowledge Translation Impacts and Implications

Insights from our study of Sudanese and Zimbabwean refugee new parents were disseminated to inform services in diverse health-related settings, as well as program and policy development that supports other refugee new parents. These vulnerable parents' experiences revealed the importance of targeted services within health systems, and coordination among agencies and organizations to mobilize support for refugee parents. The outcomes anticipated from the translation of relevant research insights include an improved cultural relevance and uptake of health interventions; an enhanced capacity of refugee new parents to manage health risks and challenges; an increased use of accessible programs to address health inequities faced by refugee families; and an expanded research and knowledge mobilization capacity relevant to vulnerable refugee parents and their children (M. Stewart, Makwarimba et al., 2015).

Building on the solid foundation of integrated knowledge transfer that involved extensive stakeholder engagement, examination of processes, and innovative and meaningful end-of-study dissemination, an online support program (developed and tested in our research) was adopted for continuation by several organizations. In the first instance, a national community agency had been a study partner (Anaphylaxis Canada, now known as Food Allergy Canada). Anaphylaxis Canada sought a license agreement with our research team to adopt the online social support-education program and learning tools developed in our funded intervention research. Parents' concerns regarding their children's isolation and health knowledge needs were alleviated by this intervention. Additional examples are illustrated in chapter 11 of other impacts on parents. The spread of new knowledge about this program is encouraging. The intended impact of integrated knowledge translation activities is the continuation and adoption of study findings in practice or public awareness to improve health outcomes.

Similarly, MOMS Link was effective in treating mothers' symptoms of postpartum depression. Findings showed that at baseline all mothers (100 per cent) were depressed, but that following approximately seven weeks of one-hour telephone calls with other mothers who experienced postpartum depression (i.e., peers), symptoms of postpartum depression were reduced to the non-clinical range for all but 8 per cent of mothers (Letourneau et al., 2015). In 2012, the program was licensed to Sykes Telecare, an original partner in the study that remained invested in the program's potential influence after study completion. As a result, the program is now available to any health region or agency by purchase from Sykes Telecare.

ATTACH™ is another such program that has been incorporated so that new agencies and professionals from health, health-related, and social service sectors may purchase training in the program from the original creators. A stakeholder from a community site where the intervention was implemented describes the significance of this:

> We have been seeing a need for attachment-based programming for the mothers in our care for a long time. We are happy that ATTACH™ can help. In fact, parents are finding ATTACH™ helps them recognize the needs of their children and how to handle situations. For example, if the child is upset and non-verbal, the mom uses ways they are taught to view the situation, and to comfort, fostering attachment.

An online learning platform has been created to train professionals to deliver this program. Currently, three agencies have ensured that their professional staff are trained to provide the ATTACH™ program independently of the research team. One agency serves vulnerable inner-city families affected by low-income, housing, and education challenges; another agency serves women and children fleeing domestic violence;

and the third agency supports Indigenous and other vulnerable women with children to overcome addictions. As one agency lead said:

> I have been a champion of ATTACH™ since the beginning and proud to offer it to our families ... ATTACH™ fills a void in the parenting programs out there by focusing on helping parents be more reflective in the relationships with their children. We have seen spectacular results.

Clearly ATTACH™ has achieved "impact at scale" by being independently delivered in the community by agencies that serve diverse, vulnerable populations.

Research that builds on the results of previous study insights through effective knowledge translation and mobilization has the potential to extend impacts into interventions with "scalability." That is, agencies that utilize research evidence in program selection may be enlisted in further validating these programs in real-world settings; testing completed interventions in more rigorous and controlled – though some might say, more artificial – settings. An Indigenous mother in one of our social support studies clearly expressed the need for using such evidence to extend the reach of programs evaluated in our intervention research:

> My biggest wish is ... if every health centre in [our region] would take one person and really seriously train them on this topic. So then they could pass on the information to the parents. Because a lot of the parents don't have the proper information or they are not sure how to give the medication. That's all I wish for.

Insights from these studies focused on varied groups of vulnerable parents (refugee, post-partum, abused, caregivers of ill children) offer innovative strategies for research and knowledge translation engaging parents facing other health inequities. Research focused on vulnerable parents is extending knowledge gained in intervention studies to inform programs and services. Integrated knowledge translation has improved health relevant outcomes and involved numerous stakeholders to maximize the impacts of research insights. Using varied engagement strategies and opportunities for dialogue, including social media, may maximize research impacts for vulnerable parents, children, families, and communities.

11 Conclusion – Insights and Implications for Future Directions

MIRIAM J. STEWART

This book interprets issues of social, economic, and cultural significance; offers insight into experiences of vulnerable children, adolescents, and parents; imparts recent research on interventions; shares scientific evidence regarding strategies for supporting children, adolescents, and families facing health inequities in Canada; and identifies implications for programs aimed at promoting health. The goals of the book identified in the introductory chapter emphasized the importance of sharing research insights regarding salient social issues; professional and experiential knowledge; intervention influences on programs and services; the lives of vulnerable children, adolescents and parents; and innovative support interventions that promote equity and inclusion. Moreover, the theoretical foundations and collaborative strategies introduced in chapter 1 guided the studies engaging with the diverse, vulnerable populations reported in this book.

Research Insights

Significant Social Issues

The diverse populations described in this book experience challenges unique to themselves, their families, and their communities. Indigenous populations face complex cultural and socio-economic challenges. Newcomers to Canada, particularly refugees, undergo both pre- and post-migration problems, with children, youth, and parents suffering mental health risks. Low-income families encounter physical and mental health problems that are exacerbated by a lack of financial resources, and financial constraints are augmented by health challenges. Families with children who have mental health conditions face uncertain futures as symptoms can influence social factors affecting children's prospects (e.g., school, employment, literacy). Parents must endure and optimally overcome risk factors and life situations affecting their health.

Many children, youth, and parents in these studies were isolated by both structural (e.g., insufficient educational and employment opportunities) and interpersonal (e.g., stereotyping, avoidance) barriers. Children, adolescents, parents, and caregivers described challenges with knowledge gaps, loneliness, and social isolation, and a lack of culturally and socio-economic appropriate support. They reported wanting to feel included, and to be able to seek support, identify their needs and capabilities, and cope with challenges.

The newcomers in our research linked formal supports, such as employment insurance and housing, to health, reflecting the importance of social determinants of health (M. Stewart, Makwarimba et al., 2010). When immigrants and refugees are thwarted in their efforts to overcome settlement challenges, they are "stuck in survival mode": unemployed, financially insecure, and struggling to improve their living situation. Differences between refugees from different countries with different cultural experiences reinforce the importance of explicating the role of ethnicity in the design of culturally relevant support intervention(s), and of offering culturally appropriate services that mobilize and sustain support (M. Stewart, Dennis et al., 2015).

Our research reports indicate that inadequate social support, social exclusion and isolation, income gaps, discrimination, institutional barriers, and policy limitations influence vulnerable children's and parents' health behaviours and use of health services.

Professional and Experiential Knowledge

Embracing both experiential knowledge of peers and the professional knowledge of health-related professionals increased understanding of life challenges, health conditions, treatment approaches, and available services. Valuing both types of knowledge also reflects the Two-eyed Seeing model, which recognizes both Western knowledge and Indigenous ways of thinking and knowing. Support from peers and professionals was essential in helping participants of all ages experience less isolation and more inclusion. Participants gained a sense of belonging and knowledge to help cope with their lives and health conditions. Refugee youth identified the importance of meeting people "they did not know before," to make friends, and be "part of a team." Low-income children with health conditions expressed appreciation for support from peers who had experiential knowledge of their conditions and life context. Service providers recognized risks, vulnerabilities, and inequities in resources; yet encountered challenges to ensuring continuity of care. Some service providers expressed "upstream" perspectives reflecting social determinants of health. They emphasized the importance of intersectoral approaches to policies and programs, preventive supports, reduction of language and cultural barriers, and enhanced access to education.

Our research also revealed the need for service providers in health and health-related sectors to appraise the economic and cultural disparities faced by vulnerable families affected by children's health inequities, and to offer accessible, relevant, and respectful supports. Some service providers seemed constrained in their ability to address health disparities by scopes of practice and prevailing policy contexts. Our studies revealed that involving service providers in support and outreach initiatives increased their understanding of vulnerable populations. Knowledge-sharing strategies should ensure that an environment of cultural humility and security is maintained. When such understanding is achieved, service providers can offer relevant support, from simple assistance to more complex actions.

Lives of Vulnerable Children, Youth, and Parents

Indigenous parents reported challenges linked to sudden and severe health crises, knowledge gaps, poverty, blame imposed for their children's illnesses, underdiagnosis, uncoordinated health care, disrespectful treatment, isolation, environmental problems, and a lack of culturally appropriate support. Refugee new parents described isolation, loneliness and stress, and cultural barriers to services and programs. Children, adolescents, and parents shared the detrimental influences of low income on the management of their health conditions, including isolation and exclusion, struggles to normalize their lives, and inadequate access to information. Poverty shaped lower-income people's perceptions of being avoided and isolated, which inhibited their involvement in community activities.

The perspectives of service providers, program planners, policy influencers, health clinic staff, family support workers, pharmacists, community health centre staff, community developers, respiratory therapists, social workers, and child/youth workers in the Canadian provinces were elicited in interviews and symposia by many of the studies shared in this book. Health service providers in our studies faced obstacles in connecting at-risk children, adolescents, and families with requisite resources, and struggled to ensure that vulnerable people receive comprehensive care. They were impeded by a lack of coordination between different systems and sectors. The information gathered from these health service providers contributed to the development of programs that could diminish health inequities and promote inclusion.

Support Interventions to Promote Inclusion and Diminish Isolation

Peer-support interventions have the potential to improve the relevance and uptake of programs informed by the needs and wishes of target populations, and to increase the efficacy of interventions through supplementing professional knowledge with credible experiential knowledge. Moreover, they enhance the capacity of children and parents to manage health constraints; improve accessibility to requisite health and community services by addressing cultural, economic, and geographic inequities; and inform the development of policies promoting the collaboration of health-related sectors. Low-income and Indigenous parents reported that they valued sharing with and learning from peers in a supportive environment.

A vital mechanism underpinning the success of many support-education projects shared in this book was enhancing accessibility. Online peer mentorship and relationship building seemed significant, particularly for geographically dispersed and isolated youth who have limited contact with others facing similar situations. The adolescents who benefited most from online support interventions previously felt excluded and isolated, suggesting the significance of targeting vulnerable youth for support interventions. Health professionals and peer mentors believed that the ability to share online in real time fostered the formation of supportive peer groups. They contended that the anonymity of the internet helped at-risk children participate in an accessible, safe meeting space. Our online support interventions are low cost and adaptable. Accordingly, they can easily be modified and replicated in diverse settings for vulnerable children, adolescents, and parents. Online support interventions also have the potential to reduce the stigma affecting low-income and Indigenous people, and children and parents from different countries of origin. Uniting with peers online could help reduce stigma through tailored services that respect the beliefs, values, and practices of unique groups.

Interventions can support coping strategies and augment protective factors associated with resilience by facilitating access to supportive resources (M. Stewart, Reid et al., 1997; Ungar, 2018). Ungar et al. (2015) found that helping youth to cope and to engage social support can be as effective as introducing formal services. The studies presented in this book reinforce the potential benefits of providing support in accessible, relevant interventions that consider risk-exposure and the fit between available resources and needs.

Influence on Programs and Services

Research can mobilize and inform service program design and development. To illustrate, a license agreement was developed between our research team and a national partner (Food Allergy Canada, formerly Anaphylaxis Canada) to adopt an online support-education program and learning tools designed and tested in our funded research. Over 95 per cent of the initial participants in the resultant programs reported satisfaction and described positive impacts on health-related outcomes including self-esteem, belonging, confidence, coping, illness management, and inclusion. By mid-2019, over 800 children and adolescents had been mentored in the Allergy Pals/Allergy Allies program offered through this partnership.

This mentorship program model has also been transferred to the Asthma Society of Canada, Camp Blue Spruce (US), Allergy and Anaphylaxis Australia, and the Eczema Society of Canada. The Asthma Society of Canada reported that successful collaborations with our research team resulted in an improved understanding of asthma and its prevention, treatment, and management. Subsequently, organizations in other countries, which had not been involved initially in the study, sought license agreements with the research team, demonstrating "scaling" internationally. To illustrate, the College of Graduate and Professional Studies at John F. Kennedy University in California acquired a license to use our research designed tools for their camp-based support program for children with food allergies and related conditions. Most recently, a license agreement was created with the National Allergy Strategy: AllergyMATE in Australia.

These successful partnerships with national and international program planners and policy influencers offered our research teams links to their networks of health professionals and other national and international organizations, and facilitated the translation and transfer of our online support-education interventions into sustainable services that benefit vulnerable children and their parents.

Conceptual Coherence and Collaborations

Consistent with theoretical foundations introduced in chapter 1, social determinants including social support, ethnicity, and income are consistently integrated through this book. Attention must also be paid to the underlying root causes of inequity (Canadian Council on Social

Determinants of Health [CCSDH], 2013). For example, increased understanding of systematic patterning of risks and resources in the social environment by race, ethnicity, and socio-economic status – and their combined influences on health outcomes (Williams et al., 2016) – is important. Indigenous peoples, community organizations, and governments are taking action to address health inequities through programs that foster education and job training, promote physical and psychological health, and strengthen community capacity. Interdisciplinary initiatives using strengths-based approaches, and collaboration with communities in true partnership, are critical for the success of research and programs in Indigenous communities. A strengths-based approach values Indigenous knowledge while integrating appropriate Western methods in culturally responsive ways. Through ethical partnerships with Indigenous communities, researchers and service providers can enable Indigenous people to identify opportunities for action and assess current gaps in resources or capacities (CCSDH, 2013). A strengths-based approach is also a salient strategy for working with refugee youth and reinforcing their resilience. Emphasizing strengths, knowledge, and abilities of youth; acknowledging the value of personal experiences; focusing on building for a positive future; and using these assets to help refugee youth cope with challenges will guide service providers in the provision of relevant support. Resilience-focused programs recognize that individuals and families at social, cultural, and economic risk can exhibit significant strength despite adversity (Mangham et al., 1996; Ungar, 2018). Interventions could encompass the education of health-related service providers regarding unique support needs and strengths of vulnerable populations.

Interdisciplinary collaboration and public participation strategies underpin the successes of our studies seeking to promote health of vulnerable children, adolescents, and families. In our experience, collaboration with multiple stakeholders ensured the relevance of research to vulnerable people, and to providers of accessible services and supports. To illustrate, our poverty-focused programs included community partners (those living in poverty and those working with low-income populations), and elicited the perspectives of policymakers and service providers (Reutter et al., 2005). Improving access to community-based services and supports for vulnerable children and families, and developing supportive programs and policies in diverse sectors would be both timely and transformative (M. Stewart, Masuda et al., 2015). Programs and policies that reduce inequalities based on income and/or ethnicity help to increase inclusion and decrease isolation (M. Stewart, Makwarimba et al., 2009). At both national and local levels, social and health programs should expand understanding of poverty, ethnicity, and their effects on vulnerable populations, and help reduce negative attitudes, interactions, and practices related to these determinants.

Implications for Future Directions

An improved understanding of why children from more disadvantaged backgrounds have worse health, and how interventions work, for whom, and in what contexts, will facilitate the reduction of inequities (Pearce et al., 2019). Diminishing inequities during early childhood necessitates a multi-faceted approach that utilizes policies to enhance access to quality social services; enables secure and flexible workplaces for parents; provides inclusive and evidence-based interventions; promotes the reinforcement of community networks; and offers timely information and support to parents (Moore et al., 2015).

While online interventions are promising, functionality, technological restrictions, design deficiencies, appropriateness, and implications for practice must all be considered (Canadian Medical Association [CMA], 2015). Our recent initiatives offer promising insights for future accessible interventions supporting low-income, immigrant, and Indigenous children and parents facing health inequities and health literacy challenges (Batterham et al., 2017). Moreover, "sharing information about programs and interventions that have been shown to reduce health inequalities contribute to the evidence base for other jurisdictions seeking to adopt similar strategies" (Canadian Institute for Health Information, 2016, p. 17).

Continuing inequalities in health linked to ethnicity and socio-economic status confirm the need for research identifying interventions at multiple societal levels that reduce and ultimately eliminate inequities in mental and physical health (Williams et al., 2016). Research is encouraged that designs and tests innovative multi-level, multi-sectoral, and multi-strategy interventions (Raphael, 2008), and that evaluates differential impacts of interventions on vulnerable population subgroups. The critical need for intersectoral strategies continues; there is a need for investment not only in health, but also in educational, economic, and social sectors to promote and protect the health of children, adolescents, and parents (Weiss & Ferrand, 2019). Partnerships engaging health service providers and stakeholders outside of traditional health care delivery roles can ensure the relevance of services to the unique needs of low-income and other vulnerable children and families (World Health Organization [WHO], 2018). Research is needed to create an evidence base that can "identify the multilevel interventions that are likely to enhance the health of all, even while they improve the health of disadvantaged groups more rapidly than the rest of the population, so that inequities in health can be reduced and ultimately eliminated" (Williams et al., 2016, p. 407).

Our studies reveal that although at-risk people encounter barriers to participation, their input is important in the development of programs, services, and policies. Community-based participatory, accessible, and acceptable support interventions are needed to meet the specific needs and wishes of vulnerable people. To reduce inequities, a collaborative approach across sectors and the effective engagement of Indigenous people, immigrants, and policy and program decision-makers are essential (CCSDH, 2013). To illustrate, Indigenous engagement in health policy design, planning, and delivery can yield more culturally responsive and accessible health care services (Lavoie et al., 2012).

Tailored programs and services acting on the needs of specific vulnerable group members (e.g., immigrant children from different countries) would be responsive to current conditions. A family-centred approach to assessment and intervention could address the complex issues facing families of children with mental (e.g., OCD) or physical (e.g., asthma) health conditions, as well as those issues facing migrant, Indigenous, and low-income families. Initiatives by service providers, clinicians, researchers, and policymakers should be integrated to decrease the burden of health conditions, and should consider the risk and protective factors that operate at individual, family, community, and population levels. Methods to achieve this goal include (1) tailored management plans to reduce the effects of social or economic adversity, and (2) connecting clients with services that help reduce social risks by increasing knowledge of risk factors (Shields-Zeeman et al., 2019). Service provider and policymaker strategies to influence social determinants of health could:

- focus on equity in practice and education; the unequal distribution of health and heath literacy; and material, psychosocial, or behavioural barriers to services access;
- generate evidence on inequalities in design, implementation, and evaluation of interventions and services, including participant representativeness and differential uptake and effectiveness;
- advocate for more equitable and child-focused resource allocation and distribution (Pearce et al., 2019); and
- remove financial barriers and consider universal approaches, including insurance- or grant-based funding, combined with directed programs that enhance equitable uptake (Mental Health Commission of Canada, 2018).

Social determinants of health influence inequities experienced by children, adolescents, and families (WHO, 2019). The Canadian government aims to reduce health inequalities and acknowledge social determinants of health by strengthening the evidence base, informing decision-making, and engaging stakeholders beyond the health sector (Government of Canada, 2018a). Proposed policy initiatives include creating a methodology to measure inequities in the guaranteed annual income approach, a national food security program, a national affordable housing program, and investment in early childhood education (Shimmin, 2015). Examining social determinants of health across age groups improves understanding of the influences of early life socio-economic status and other diversity modes, including health literacy, on adult health inequities (Poureslami et al., 2017; Williams et al., 2016).

Interventions aimed at reducing economic inequalities should also address the additional effects of ethnicity (Williams et al., 2016) and gender (Hilario et al., 2014). To improve underlying social and economic factors that lead to health disparities, the Canadian government must acknowledge differences in access and quality of care for many groups (CMA, 2017).

Throughout this book, salient social determinants of health introduced in the initial chapter – social support, socio-economic status, ethnicity, and gender – guide each chapter's content. Primary principles – diversity of support providers and recipients, multiplicity of supporters and supported, equity and egalitarianism, reciprocity in support exchange – are depicted on the book's cover. Vulnerable children, adolescents, and caregivers, including people of low income, Indigenous people, immigrants, and refugees, are the focus of diverse support interventions targeted to their specific needs and preferences.

References

Abbey, R.D., Clopton, J.R., & Humphreys, J.D. (2007). Obsessive-compulsive disorder and romantic functioning. *Journal of Clinical Psychology, 63*(12), 1181–92. https://doi.org/10.1002/jclp.20423. Medline:17972290

Abidi, S. (2017). Paving the way to change for youth at the gap between child and adolescent and adult mental health services. *Canadian Journal of Psychiatry, 62*(6), 388–92. https://doi.org/10.1177/0706743717694166. Medline:28562089

Aboriginal Nurses Association of Canada. (2014). Capacity building for leadership in health care governance and management. Aboriginal Nurses Association of Canada.

Ahmed, S.M., Beck, B., Maurana, C.A. & Newton, G. (2004). Overcoming barriers to effective community-based participatory research in US medical schools. *Education for Health, 17*(2), 141–51. https://doi.org/10.1080/13576280410001710969. Medline:15763757

Alaazi, D.A., Salami, B., Yohani, S., Vallianatos, H., Okeke-Ihejirika, P., & Nsaliwa, C. (2018). Transnationalism, parenting, and child disciplinary practices of African immigrants in Alberta, Canada. *Child Abuse & Neglect, 86*, 147–57. https://doi.org/10.1016/j.chiabu.2018.013. Medline:30292095

Alavi, N., Roberts, N., & DeGrace, E. (2017). Comparison of parental socio-demographic factors in children and adolescents presenting with internalizing and externalizing disorders. *International Journal of Adolescent Medicine & Health, 29*(2), 41. https://doi.org/10.1515/ijamh-2015-0049. Medline:26418644

Alegría, M., NeMoyer, A., Falgàs Bagué, I., Wang, Y., & Alvarez, K. (2018). Social determinants of mental health: Where we are and where we need to go. *Current Psychiatry Reports, 20*(11), 95. https://doi.org/10.1007/s11920-018-0969-9. Medline:30221308

Alemany-Navarro, M., Costas, J., Real, E., Segalàs, C., Bertolín, S., Domènech, L., Rabionet, R., Carracedo, A., Menchón, J.M., & Alonso, P. (2019).

Do polygenic risk and stressful life events predict pharmacological treatment response in obsessive compulsive disorder? A gene-environment interaction approach. *Translational Psychiatry, 9*(1), 70. https://doi.org/10.1038 /s41398-019-0410-0. Medline:30718812

Ali, J. (2002). *Mental health of Canada's Immigrants. Supplement to Health Reports, 13.* Statistics Canada, Cat. no. 82-003.

Allan, B., & Smylie, J. (2015). *First Peoples, second class treatment: The role of racism in the health and well-being of Indigenous peoples in Canada.* The Wellesley Institute. https://www.wellesleyinstitute.com/wp-content /uploads/2015/02/Summary-First-Peoples-Second-Class-Treatment-Final .pdf

Alvarenga, P.G., do Rosario, M.C., Cesar, R.C., Manfro, G.G., Moriyama, T.S., Bloch, M.H., Shavitt, R.G., Hoexter, M.Q., Coughlin, C.G., Leckman, J.F., & Miguel, E.C. (2016). Obsessive-compulsive symptoms are associated with psychiatric comorbidities, behavioral and clinical problems: a population-based study of Brazilian school children. *European Child & Adolesccent Psychiatry, 25*(2), 175–82. https://doi.org/10.1007/s00787-015-0723-3. Medline:26015374

American Psychiatric Association. (2013). *Diagnostic and statistical manual of mental disorders* (5th ed.). American Psychiatric Association.

Amir, N., Freshman, M., & Foa, E.B. (2000). Family distress and involvement in relatives of obsessive-compulsive disorder patients. *Journal of Anxiety Disorders, 14*(3), 209–17. https://doi.org/10.1016/S0887-6185(99)00032-8. Medline:10868980

Amthor, R.F., & Roxas, K. (2016). Multicultural education and newcomer youth: Re-imagining a more inclusive vision for immigrant and refugee students. *Education Studies, 52*(2), 155–76. https://doi.org/10.1080/00131946 .2016.1142992

Andermann, A. (2016). Taking action on the social determinants of health in clinical practice: A framework for health professionals. *Canadian Medical Association Journal, 188*(17–18), E474–83. https://doi.org/10.1503/cmaj .160177. Medline:27503870

Anderson, L.M., Freeman, J.B., Franklin, M.E., & Sapyta, J.J. (2015). Family-based treatment of pediatric obsessive-compulsive disorder: Clinical considerations and application. *Child & Adolescent Psychiatric Clinics of North America, 24*(3), 535–55. https://doi.org/10.1016/j.chc.2015.02.003. Medline:26092738

Andersson, N., & Ledogar, R.J. (2008). The CIET Aboriginal youth resilience studies: 14 years of capacity building and methods development in Canada. *Pimatisiwin, 6*(2), 65–88. Medline:20862230

Andrighetti, H., Semaka, A., Stewart, S.E., Shuman, C., Hayeems, R., & Austin, J. (2016). Obsessive-compulsive disorder: The process of parental adaptation and implications for genetic counseling. *Journal of Genetic Counseling, 25*(5), 912–22. https://doi.org/10.1007/s10897-015-9914-9. Medline:26639756

Angus Reid Institute. (2015). *Prescription drug access and affordability an issue for nearly a quarter of all Canadian households.* http://angusreid.org/wp-content /uploads/2015/07/2015. 07.09Pharma.pdf

Anholt, G.E., Aderka, I.M., van Balkom, A.J., Smit, J.H., Schruers, K., van der Wee, N.J., Eikelenboom, M., De Luca, V., & van Oppen, P. (2013). Age of onset in obsessive-compulsive disorder: admixture analysis with a large sample. *Psychological Medicine, 44*(1), 185–94. https://doi.org/10.1017 /S0033291713000470. Medline:23517651

Anisef, P., Brown, R. S., Phythian, K., Sweet, R., & Walters, D. (2010). Early school leaving among immigrants in Toronto secondary schools. *Canadian Review of Sociology, 47*(2), 103–28. https://doi.org/10.1111/j.1755-618x .2010.01226.x. Medline:20853810

Aspvall, K., Andrén, P., Lenhard, F., Andersson, E., Mataix-Cols, D., & Serlachius, E. (2018). Internet-delivered cognitive behavioural therapy for young children with obsessive-compulsive disorder: development and initial evaluation of the BIP OCD Junior programme. *BJPsych Open, 4*(3), 106–12. https://doi.org/10.1192/bjo.2018.10. Medline:29971153

Assembly of First Nations. (2007). *First Nations regional longitudinal health survey: Our voice, our survey, our reality. Selected results from RHS phase 1 (2002/03).* Assembly of First Nations.

Asthma Society of Canada (ASC). (2014). *Severe asthma: The Canadian patient journey.* Asthma Society of Canada. https://asthma.ca/wp-content/uploads /2017/06/SAstudy.pdf

Atkinson, D. (2017). *Considerations for Indigenous child and youth population mental health promotion in Canada.* National Collaborating Centres for Public Health.

Azzopardi, P.S., Hearps, S.J.C., Francis, K.L., Kennedy, E.C., Mokdad, A.H., Kassebaum, N.J., Lim, S., Irvine, C.M.S., Vos, T., Brown, A.D., Dogra, S., Kinner, S.A., Kaoma, N.S., Naguib, M., Reavley, N.J., Requejo, J., Santelli, J.S., Sawyer, S.M., Skirbekk, V., Temmerman, M., Tewhaiti-Smith, J., Ward, J.L., Viner, R.M., & Patton, G.C. (2019). Progress in adolescent health and wellbeing: Tracking 12 headline indicators for 195 countries and territories, 1990–2016. *Lancet, 393*, 1101–18. https://doi.org/10.1016/S0140-6736(18)32427-9. Medline:30876706

Baker-Ericzen, M.J., Jenkins, M.M., & Haine-Schlagel, R. (2013). Therapist, parent, and youth perspectives of treatment barriers to family-focused community outpatient mental health services. *Journal of Child & Family Studies, 22*(6), 854–68. https://doi.org/10.1007/s10826-012-9644-7. Medline:24019737

Banulescu-Bogdan, N. (2020). *Beyond work: Reducing social isolation for refugee women and other marganized newcomers.* Migration Policy Institute.

Bartlett, C., Marshall, M., & Marshall, A. (2012). Two-Eyed Seeing and other lessons learned within a co-learning journey of bringing together indigenous and mainstream knowledges and ways of knowing. *Journal of Environmental Studies & Sciences, 2*(4), 86–8. https://doi.org/10.1007 /s13412-012-0086-8

Bartram, M. (2019). Income-based inequities in access to mental health services in Canada. *Canadian Journal of Public Health, 110*(4), 395–403. https://doi .org/10.17269/s41997-019-00204-5. Medline:30989633

Barzilay, R., Patrick, A., Calkins, M.E., Moore, T.M., Wolf, D.H., Benton, T.D., Leckman, J.F., Gur, R.C., & Gur, R.E. (2019). Obsessive-compulsive symptomatology in community youth: Typical development or a red flag for psychopathology? *Journal of the American Academy of Child & Adolescent Psychiatry, 58*(2), 277–86.e274. https://doi.org/10.1016/j.jaac.2018.06.038. Medline:30738554

Batterham, R.W., Beauchamp, A., & Osborne, R.H. (2017). Health literacy. In S.R. Quah (Ed.), *International Encyclopedia of Public Health* (2nd ed., pp. 428–37). Academic Press. doi.org/10.1016/B978-0-12-803678-5.00190-9.

Beck, A., Nadkarni, A., Calam, R., Naeem, F., & Husain, N. (2016). Increasing access to cognitive behaviour therapy in low and middle income countries: A strategic framework. *Asian Journal of Psychiatry, 22*, 190–5. https://doi.org /10.1016/j.ajp.2015.10.008. Medline:26643366

Becker, M., Mishra, S., Aral, S., Bhattacharjee, P., Lorway, R., Green, K., Anthony, J., Isac, S., Emmanuel, F., Musyoki, H., Lazarus, L., Thompson, L. H., Cheuk, E., & Blanchard, J. F. (2018). The contributions and future direction of Program Science in HIV/STI prevention. *Emerging Themes Epidemiology, 15*, 1–7. https://doi.org/10.1186/s12982-018-0076-8. Medline:29872450

Beiser, M., Goodwill, A.M., Albanese, P., McShane, K., & Nowakowski, M. (2014). Predictors of immigrant children's mental health in Canada: Selection, settlement contingencies, culture, or all of the above? *Social Psychiatry and Psychiatric Epidemiology, 49*(5), 743–56. https://doi.org /10.1007/s00127-013-0794-8. Medline:24318040

Beiser, M., Hamilton, H., Rummens, J.A., Oxman-Martinez, J., Ogilvie, L., Humphrey, C., & Armstrong, R. (2010). Predictors of emotional problems and physical aggression among children of Hong Kong Chinese, Mainland Chinese and Filipino immigrants to Canada. *Social Psychiatry and Psychiatric Epidemiology, 45*(10), 1011–21. https://doi.org/10.1007/s00127-009-0140-3. Medline:19768355

Beiser, M., Hou, F., Hyman, I., & Tousignant, M. (2002). Poverty, family process, and the mental health of immigrant children in Canada. *American Journal of Public Health, 92*(2), 220–7. https://doi.org/10.2105/ajph.92.2.220. Medline:11818295

Beiser, M., & Stewart, S. (2005). Reducing health disparities: A priority for Canada (Preface). *Canadian Journal of Public Health, 96*(S2), S4–S5.

Beiser, M., Taa, B., Fenta-Wube, H., Baheretibeb, Y., Pain, C., & Araya, M. (2012). A comparison of levels and predictors of emotional problems among preadolescent Ethiopians in Addis Ababa, Ethiopia, and Toronto, Canada. *Transcultural Psychiatry, 49*(5), 651–77. https://doi.org/10.1177/1363461512457155. Medline:23015641

Beiser, M., Zilber, N., Simich, L., Youngmann, R., Zohar, A.H., Taa, B., & Hou, F. (2011). Regional effects on the mental health of immigrant children: Results from the new Canadian children and youth study (NCCYS). *Health and Place, 17*(3), 822–9. https://doi.org/10.1016/j.healthplace.2011.03.005. Medline:21463966

Belhadj Kouider, E., Koglin, U. & Petermann, F. (2015). Emotional and behavioral problems in migrant children and adolescents in American countries: A systematic review. *Journal of Immigrant and Minority Health, 17*(4), 1240–58. https://doi.org/10.1007/s1090. Medline:24851820

Belschner, L., Lin, S.Y., Yamin, D.F., Best, J., Edalati, K., McDermid, J., & Stewart, S.E. (2020). Mindfulness-based skills training group for parents of obsessive-compulsive disorder affected children: A caregiver focused intervention. *Complementary Therapies in Clinical Practice, 39*, 101098. https://doi.org/10.1016/j.ctcp.2020.101098

Benedetti, F., Poletti, S., Radaelli, D., Pozzi, E., Giacosa, C., & Smeraldi, E. (2014). Adverse childhood experiences and gender influence treatment seeking behaviors in obsessive-compulsive disorder. *Comprehensive Psychiatry, 55*(2), 298–301. https://doi.org/10.1016/j.comppsych.2013.08.028. Medline:24262116

Bergold, J., & Thomas, S. (2012). Participatory research methods: A methodological approach in motion. *Historical Social Research, 37*(4), 191–222. https://www.jstor.org/stable/41756482

Berkes, F. (2009). Indigenous ways of knowing and the study of environmental change. *Journal of the Royal Society of New Zealand, 39*(4), 151–6. https://doi.org/10.1080/03014220909510568

Berry, J., & Hou, F. (2016). Immigration acculturation and well-being in Canada. *Canadian Psychology, 57*(4), 254–64. https://doi.org/10.1037/cap0000064

Blais, L., Beauchesne, M-F., & Levesque, S. (2006). Socioeconomic status and medication prescription patterns in pediatric asthma in Canada. *Journal of Adolescent Health, 38*(5), e9–16. https://doi.org/10.1016/j.jadohealth.2005.02.010. Medline:16635775

Bloch, M.H., Craiglow, B.G., Landeros-Weisenberger, A., Dombrowski, P.A., Panza, K.E., Peterson, B.S., & Leckman, J.F. (2009). Predictors of early adult outcomes in pediatric-onset obsessive-compulsive disorder.

Pediatrics, 124(4), 1085–93. https://doi.org/10.1542/peds.2009-0015. Medline:19786445

Block, S., Galabuzi, G.E., & Tranjan, R. (2019). Canada's colour coded income inequality. *Canadian Centre for Policy Alternatives.*

Blom, M.M., Bosmans, J.E., Cuijpers, P., Zarit, S.H., & Pot, A.M. (2013). Effectiveness and cost-effectiveness of an internet intervention for family caregivers of people with dementia: Design of a randomized controlled trial. *BMC Psychiatry, 13*(1), 17. https://doi.org/10.1186/1471-244X-13-17. Medline:23305463

Blom, M.M., Zarit, S.H., Zwaaftink, R.B.G., Cuijpers P., & Pot, A.M. (2015). Effectiveness of an internet intervention for family caregivers of people with dementia: Results of a randomized controlled trial. *PLoS One, 10*(2). https://doi.org/10.1371/journal.pone.0116622. Medline:25679228

Bøe, T., Sivertsen, B., Heiervang, E., Goodman, R., Lundervold, A.J., & Hysing, M. (2014). Socioeconomic status and child mental health: The role of parental emotional well-being and parenting practices. *Journal of Abnormal Child Psychology, 42*(5), 705–15. https://doi.org/10.1007/s10802-013 -9818-9. Medline:24150864

Boffa, J., King, M., McMullin, K., & Long, R. (2011). A process for the inclusion of Aboriginal people in health research: Lessons from the Determinants of TB Transmission Project. *Social Science and Medicine, 72*(5), 733–8. https://doi .org/10.1016/j.socscimed.2010.10.033. Medline:21316828

Bolatova, T., & Law, M. (2019). Income-related disparities in private prescription drug coverage in Canada. *CMAJ Open, 7*(4). https://doi.org /10.9778.cmajo.20190085. Medline:31604712

Boots, L.M., de Vugt, M.E., van Knippenberg, R.J., Kempen, G.I., & Verhey, F.R. (2014). A systematic review of internet-based supportive interventions for caregivers of patients with dementia. *International Journal of Geriatric Psychiatry, 29*(4), 331–44. https://doi.org/10.1002/gps.4016. Medline:23963684

Borkman, T. (1999). *Understanding self-help/mutual aid: Experiential learning in the commons.* George Mason University.

Bourque, F.I., van der Ven, E., & Malla, A. (2011). A meta-analysis of the risk for psychotic disorders among first- and second-generation immigrants. *Psychological Medicine, 41*(5), 897–910. https://doi.org/10.1017/S0033291710001406. Medline:20663257

Bourque Bearskin, L., Kennedy, Bourque, D., Bourque, D.H., & Cardinal, S. (2020). Nursing leadership in indigenous health. In P. Yoder-Wise, J. Waddell, & N. Walton (Eds.), *Leading and managing in Canadian nursing* (2nd ed., pp. 54–84). Elsevier.

Bourque Bearskin, R. L., Kennedy, A., Kelly, L., & Chakanyuka, C. (2021). Indigenous nursing: Caring keeps us close to the source. In M. Hills,

J. Watson, & C. Cara (Eds.) *Creating a caring science curriculum: An emancipatory pedagogy for nursing* (pp. 249–70). Springer.

Boyle, M.H., Georgiades, K., Duncan, L., Wang, L., & Comeau, J. (2019). Poverty, neighbourhood antisocial behaviour, and children's mental health problems: Findings from the 2014 Ontario Child Health Study. *Canadian Journal of Psychiatry, 64*(4), 285–93. https://doi.org/10.1177/0706743719830027. Medline:30978142

Boyle, M.H., & Lipman, E.L. (2002). Do places matter? Socioeconomic disadvantage and behavioral problems of children in Canada. *Journal of Consulting and Clinical Psychology, 70*(2), 378–89. https://doi.org/10.1037//0022-006x.70.2.378. Medline:11952196

Bradley, R.H., & Corwyn, R.F. (2002). Socioeconomic status and child development. *Annual Review of Psychology, 53*, 371–99. https://doi.org/10.1146/annurev.psych.53.100901.135233

Brander, G., Rydell, M., Kuja-Halkola, R., Fernández de la Cruz, L., Lichtenstein, P., Serlachius, E., Rück, C., Almqvist, C., D'Onofrio, B.M., Larsson, H., & Mataix-Cols, D. (2016). Association of perinatal risk factors with obsessive-compulsive disorder: A population-based birth cohort, sibling control study. *JAMA Psychiatry, 73*(11), 1135–44. https://doi.org/10.1001/jamapsychiatry.2016.2095. Medline:27706475

Brauer, L., Lewin, A.B., & Storch, E.A. (2011). Evidence-based treatment for pediatric obsessive-compulsive disorder. *Israel Journal of Psychiatry & Related Sciences, 48*(4), 280–7. Medline:22572092

Brave Heart, M.Y.H., Chase, J., Elkins, J., & Altshul, D.B. (2011). Historical trauma among Indigenous peoples of the Americas: Concepts, research, and clinical considerations. *Journal of Psychoactive Drugs, 43*(4), 282–90. https://doi.org/10.1080/02791072.2011.628913. Medline:22400458

Brent, D.A. (2020). Commentary: Reducing adolescent suicide: a global imperative – a reflection on Glenn et al. (2020). *Journal of Child Psychology & Psychiatry, 61*(3), 309–11. https://doi.org/10.1111/jcpp.13174. Medline:31820433

Briggs, E.S., & Price, I.R. (2009). The relationship between adverse childhood experience and obsessive-compulsive symptoms and beliefs: The role of anxiety, depression, and experiential avoidance. *Journal of Anxiety Disorders, 23*(8), 1037–46. https://doi.org/10.1016/j.janxdis.2009.07.004. Medline:19635653

Bronstein, I., & Montgomery, P. (2011). Psychological distress in refugee children: A systematic review. *Clinical, Child and Family Psychology, 14*(1), 44–56. https://doi.org/10.1007/s10567-010-0081-0. Medline:21181268

Browne, A.J. (2017). Moving beyond description: Closing the health equity gap by redressing racism impacting Indigenous populations. *Social Science and Medicine, 184*, 23–6. https://doi.org/10.1016/j.socscimed.2017.04.045. Medline:28494318

Browne, A.J., Varcoe, C., Lavoie, J., Smye, V., Wong, S.T., Krause, M., Tu, D., Godwin, O., Khan, K., & Fridkin, A. (2016). Enhancing health care equity with Indigenous populations: Evidence-based strategies from an ethnographic study. *BMC Health Services Research, 16*, 544. https://doi.org/10.1186/s12913-016-1707-9

Calati, R., Ferrari, C., Brittner, M., Oasi, O., Olié, E., Carvalho, A.F., & Courtet, P. (2018). Suicidal thoughts and behaviors and social isolation: A narrative review of the literature. *Journal of Affective Disorders, 245*, 653–67. https://doi.org/10.1016/j.jad.2018.11.022. Medline:30445391

Calvocoressi, L., Lewis, B., Harris, M., Trufan, S.J., Goodman, W.K., McDougle, C.J., & Price, L.H. (1995). Family accommodation in obsessive-compulsive disorder. *American Journal of Psychiatry, 152*(3), 441–3. https://doi.org/10.1176/ajp.152.3.441

Canadian Council of Child and Youth Advocates. (2011). *Aboriginal children: Canada must do better: Today and tomorrow.* http://provincialadvocate.on.ca/documents/en/CCCYA_UN_Report.pdf

Canadian Council on Social Determinants of Health (CCSDH). (2013). *Roots of resilience: Overcoming inequities in Aboriginal Communities.* http://ccsdh.ca/images/uploads/Roots_of_Resilience.pdf

Canadian Institute for Health Information (CIHI). (2016). *Trends in income-related health inequalities in Canada: Technical report.* https://secure.cihi.ca/free_products/trends_in_income_related_inequalities_in_canada_2015_en.pdf?_ga=2.115633358.938938568.1560190695-1741887880.1548291742

Canadian Institute for Health Information (CIHI). (2018). *Asthma hospitalizations among children and youth in Canada: Trends and inequalities.* www.cihi.ca/sites/default/files/document/asthma-hospitalization-children-2018-chartbook-en-web.pdf

Canadian Institutes of Health Research (CIHR). (2013). *Internal assessment for 2011 international review – CIHR Institute of Aboriginal Peoples' Health.* http://www.cihr-irsc.gc.ca/e/43686.html

Canadian Institutes of Health Research (CIHR). (2017). CheckUp: Time to focus on and learning from Inuit (CIHR Project). *Funding decisions database – Detailed information.* http://webapps.cihr-irsc.gc.ca/decisions/p/project_details.html?applId=372682&lang=en

Canadian Institutes of Health Research (CIHR). (2018). Deepening the roots of living in a good way for Indigenous Children: The Indigenous Youth Mentorship Program (CIHR Pathways Implementation Research). *Funding decisions database – Detailed information.* http://webapps.cihr-irsc.gc.ca/decisions/p/project_details.html?applId=391922&lang=en

Canadian Institutes of Health Research (CIHR). (2019). *Strategy for patient-oriented research.* http://www.cihr-irsc.gc.ca/e/41204.html

Canadian Medical Association (CMA). (2015). *Guiding principles for physicians recommending mobile health applications to patients.* CMA Policy Statements. https://policybase.cma.ca/en/permalink/policy11521

Canadian Medical Association (CMA). (2017). *CMA submission: CMA's recommendations for effective poverty reduction strategies.* Submission to the House of Commons Standing Committee on Human Resources, Skills and Social Development and the Status of Persons with Disabilities. https://policybase.cma.ca/en

Canadian Nurses Association (CNA). (2014a). *Aboriginal health nursing and Aboriginal health: Charting policy direction for nursing in Canada.* Canadian Nurses Association.

Canadian Nurses Association (CNA). (2014b). *Why we are worried: The facts – First Nations, Inuit and Métis health.* [Fact sheet]. National Expert Commission. www.cna-aiic.ca/~/media/cna/files/en/fact_sheet_07_e.pdf?la=en

Canadian Public Health Association. (2018, December 17). *Racism and public health.* www.cpha.ca/racism-and-public-health

Cappa, C., & Giulivi, S. (2019). Adolescence and social determinants of health: Family and community. In A. Pingitore, F. Mastorci, & C. Vassalle (Eds.), *Adolescent health and wellbeing: Current strategies and future trends* (pp. 205–29). Springer. https://doi.org/10.1007/978-3-030-25816-0_10

Cargo, M., & Mercer, S.L. (2008). The value and challenges of participatory research: Strengthening its practice. *Annual Review of Public Health, 29,* 325–50. https://doi.org/10.1146/annurev.publhealth.29.091307.083824. Medline:18173388

Caron, J., & Liu, A. (2010). A descriptive study of the prevalence of psychological distress and mental disorders in the Canadian population: Comparison between low-income and non-low-income populations. *Chronic Diseases in Canada, 30*(3), 84–94. Medline:20609292

Carrière, G.M., Garner, R., & Sanmartin, C. (2017). Housing conditions and respiratory hospitalizations among first nations people in Canada. *Health Reports, 28*(4), 9–15. https://www.scopus.com/inward/record.uri?eid=2-s2.0-85018327072&partnerID=40&md5=f2e0e5a35a2ac668d8a6eed7fe61d1f7

Carver, J., Cappelli, M., & Davidson, S. (2015). Taking the next step forward: Building a responsive mental health and addictions system for emerging adults. *Mental Health Commission of Canada.* www.mentalhealthcommission.ca/English/issues/child-and-youth/taking-next-step-forward

Cassidy, J., & Asher, S. (1992). Loneliness and peer relations in young children. *Child Development, 63*(2), 350–65. https://doi.org/10.1111/j.1467-8624.1992.tb01632.x. Medline:1611939

Caxaj, C.S., Schill, K., & Janke, R. (2018). Priorities and challenges for a palliative approach to care for rural indigenous populations: A scoping review. *Health & Social Care in the Community, 26*(3), e336. https://doi.org /10.1111/hsc.12469. Medline:28703394

Centers for Disease Control and Prevention (CDCP). (2019a). Adverse childhood experiences. https://www.cdc.gov/violenceprevention /childabuseandneglect/acestudy

Centers for Disease Control and Prevention (CDCP). (2019b). Health-related quality of life. https://www.cdc.gov/hrqol/concept.htm

Chambless, D.L., Floyd, F.J., Rodebaugh, T.L., & Steketee, G.S. (2007). Expressed emotion and familial interaction: A study with agoraphobic and obsessive-compulsive patients and their relatives. *Journal of Abnormal Psychology, 116*(4), 754–61. https://doi.org/10.1037/0021-843X.116.4.754. Medline:18020721

Chandler, M.J., & Lalonde, C. (1998). Cultural continuity as a hedge against suicide in Canada's First Nations. *Transcultural Psychiatry, 35*(2), 191–219. https://doi.org/10.1177/136346159803500202

Chang, H., Beach, J., & Senthilselvan, A. (2012). Prevalence of and risk factors for asthma in off-reserve Aboriginal children and adults in Canada. *Canadian Respiratory Journal, 19*(6), e68–74. https://doi.org/10.1155/2012/753040. Medline:23248805

Cherian, A.V., Pandian, D., Math, S.B., Kandavel, T., & Janardhan Reddy, Y.C. (2014). Family accommodation of obsessional symptoms and naturalistic outcome of obsessive-compulsive disorder. *Psychiatry Research, 215*(2), 372–8. https://doi.org/10.1016/j.psychres.2013.11.017. Medline:24368062

Chibucos, T.R., Leite, R.W., & Weis, D.L. (2005). Social exchange theory. In T.R. Chibucos, R.W. Leite, & D.L. Weis (Eds.), *Readings in family theory* (pp. 137–9). Sage Publications.

Chong, S.A., Abdin, E., Picco, L., Pang, S., Jeyagurunathan, A., Vaingankar, J. A., Kwok, K.W., & Subramaniam, M. (2016). Recognition of mental disorders among a multiracial population in Southeast Asia. *BMC Psychiatry, 16*(1), 121. https://doi.org/10.1186/s12888-016-0837-2. Medline:27142577

Choo, E.K., Ranney, M.L., Chan, T.M., Trueger, N.S., Walsh, A.E., Tegtmeyer, K., McNamara, S.O., Choi, R.Y., & Carroll, C.L. (2015). Twitter as a tool for communication and knowledge exchange in academic medicine: A guide for skeptics and novices. *Medical Teacher, 37*(5), 411–16. https://doi.org/10 .3109/0142159X.2014.993371. Medline:25523012

Chrismas, B., & Chrismas, B. (2017). Social innovation narratives: What are we doing to protect newcomer youth in Canada, and help them succeed? *Journal of Community Safety & Well-Being, 2*(3). https://journalcswb.ca/index.php /cswb/article/view/52/112

Chu, B.C., Colognori, D.B., Yang, G., Xie, M.G., Lindsey Bergman, R., & Piacentini, J. (2015). Mediators of exposure therapy for youth obsessive-compulsive disorder: specificity and temporal sequence of client and treatment factors. *Behavior Therapy, 46*(3), 395–408. https://doi.org/10.1016 /j.beth.2015.01.003. Medline:25892174

Citizens for Public Justice (CPJ). (2018). *Poverty trends 2018*. www.cpj.ca /poverty-trends-2018

Citizenship and Immigration Canada. (2009). *Facts and Figures – Immigration overview: Permanent and temporary residents 2008*. www.cic.gc.ca/english/pdf /research-stats/facts2008.pdf

Citizenship and Immigration Canada. (2016). Canada – Permanent residents by immigration category, 1980-Q1 2016. [Immigrant, Refugees and Citizenship Canada, 31 March 2016 Data]. http://open.canada.ca/data /en/dataset/ad975a26-df23-456a-8ada-756191a23695?_ga=1.113254087 .1178150052.1467642374

CityNews (2016, September). African-Canadians unfairly treated by Ontario's child-welfare system: report. https://toronto.citynews.ca/2016/09/29 /african-canadians-unfairly-treated-ontarios-child-welfare-system-report/

Codjoe, H.M. (2001). Fighting 'public enemy' of black academic achievement – the persistence of racism and the schooling experiences of black students in Canada. *Race Ethnicity & Education, 4*(4), 343–75. https://doi .org/10.1080/13613320120096652

Cohen, G.L., Garcia, J., Apfel, N., & Master, A. (2006). Reducing the racial achievement gap: A social-psychological intervention. *Science, 313*(5791), 1307–10. https://doi.org/10.1126/science.1128317. Medline:16946074

Cohn, L.N., Pechlivanoglou, P., Lee, Y., Mahant, S., Orkin, J., Marson, A., & Cohen, E. (2020). Health outcomes of parents of children with chronic illness: A systematic review and meta-analysis. *The Journal of Pediatrics, 218*, 166–77.e2. https://doi.org/10.1016/jpeds.2019.10.068

Comer, J.S., Furr, J.M., Kerns, C.E., Miguel, E., Coxe, S., Elkins, R.M., Carpenter, A.L., Cornacchio, D., Cooper-Vince, C.E., DeSerisy, M., Chou, T., Sanchez, A.L., Khanna, M., Franklin, M.E., Garcia, A.M., & Freeman, J.B. (2017). Internet-delivered, family-based treatment for early-onset OCD: A pilot randomized trial. *Journal of Consulting & Clinical Psychology, 85*(2), 178–86. https://doi.org/10.1037/ccp0000155. Medline:27869451

Commission on Social Determinants of Health (CSDH). (2008). *Closing the gap in a generation: Health equity through action on the social determinants of health – Final report of the Commission on Social Determinants of Health*. World Health Organization.

Community Foundations of Canada. (2010). *Canada's vital signs 2010*. www .vitalsignscanada.ca/pdf/2010_researchfindings.pdf

Coombes, J., Hunter, K., Mackean, T., Holland, A.J.A., Sullivan, E., & Ivers, R. (2018). Factors that impact access to ongoing health care for First Nation children with a chronic condition. *BMC Health Services Research, 18*(448). https://doi.org/10.1186/s12913-018-3263-y. Medline:29898727

Cooper, M. (1996). Obsessive-compulsive disorder: Effects on family members. *American Journal of Orthopsychiatry, 66*(2), 296–304. https://doi.org/10.1037/h0080180. Medline:8860758

Costello, E.J., Angold, A., Burns, B.J., Stangl, D.K., Tweed, D.L., Erkanli, A., & Worthman, C.M. (1996). The Great Smoky Mountains Study of youth: Goals, design, methods, and the prevalence of DSM-III-R disorders. *Archives of General Psychiatry, 53*(12), 1129–36. https://doi.org/10.1001/archpsyc.1996.01830120067012. Medline:8956679

Creese, G., & Wiebe, B. (2012). 'Survival employment': Gender and deskilling among African immigrants in Canada. *International Migration, 50*(5), 56–76. https://doi.org/10.1111/j.1468-2435.2009.00531.x

Crighton, E.J., Wilson, K., & Senécal, S. (2010). The relationship between geographic and socioeconomic factors and asthma among Canada's Aboriginal populations: An analysis of the 2001 Aboriginal People's Survey. *International Journal of Circumpolar Health, 69*(2), 138–50. https://doi.org/10.3402/ijch.v69i2.17435. Medline:20356468

Crombie, I.K., Irvine, L., Elliott, L., & Wallace, H. (2005). *Closing the health inequalities gap: An international perspective.* WHO Regional Office for Europe.

Cromer, K.R., Schmidt, N.B., & Murphy, D.L. (2007). An investigation of traumatic life events and obsessive-compulsive disorder. *Behaviour Research & Therapy, 45*(7), 1683–91. https://doi.org/10.1016/j.brat.2006.08.018. Medline:17067548

Crowshoe, L., Dannenbaum, D., Green, M., Henderson, R., Naqshbandi Hayward, M., & Toth, E. (2018). Type 2 diabetes and Indigenous peoples. *Canadian Journal of Diabetes, 42*, S296–S306. https://doi.org/10.1016/j.jcjd.2017.10.022. Medline:29650108

Currie, C.L., Wild, T.C., Schopflocher, D.P., Laing, L., & Veugelers, P. (2012). Racial discrimination experienced by Aboriginal university students in Canada. *Canadian Journal of Psychiatry, 57*(10), 617–25. https://doi.org/10.1177/070674371205701006. Medline:23072953

Dahl, R.E. (2007). Sleep and the developing brain. *Sleep, 30*(9), 1079–80. https://doi.org/10.1093/sleep/30.9.1079

Dam, A.H.D., van Boxtel, M.P.J., Rozendaal, N., Verhey, F.R.J., & de Vugt, M.E. (2017). Development and feasibility of Inlife: A pilot study of an online social support intervention for informal caregivers of people with dementia. *PloS one.* https://doi.org/10.1371/journal.pone.0183386. Medline:28886056

Danso, R. (2002). From 'there' to 'here': An investigation of the initial settlement experiences of Ethiopian and Somali refugees in Toronto. *GeoJournal, 56*(1), 3–14. https://doi.org/10.1023/A:10217487

David, W. (Ed.). (1999). *Network exchange theory.* Praeger.

Davies, J.S. (2005). The social exclusion debate: Strategies, controversies and dilemmas. *Policy Studies, 26*(1), 3–27. https://doi.org/10.1080/01442870500041561

Deatrick, J. (2017). Where is "family" in the social determinants of health? Implications for family nursing practice, research, education, and policy [editorial]. *Journal of Family Nursing, 23*(4), 423–33. https://doi.org/10.1177/1074840717735287. Medline:29046117

De Luca, V., Gershenzon, V., Burroughs, E., Javaid, N., & Richter, M.A. (2011). Age at onset in Canadian OCD patients: Mixture analysis and systematic comparison with other studies. *Journal of Affective Disorders, 133*(1–2), 300–4. https://doi.org/10.1016/j.jad.2011.03.041. Medline:21546093

Denys, D., Burger, H., van Megen, H., de Geus, F., & Westenberg, H. (2003). A score for predicting response to pharmacotherapy in obsessive-compulsive disorder. *International Clinical Psychopharmacology, 18*(6), 315–22. https://doi.org/10.1097/00004850-200311000-00002. Medline:14571151

Donnelly, T.T., Hwang, J.J., Este, D., Ewashen, C., Adair, C., & Clinton, M. (2011). If I was going to kill myself, I wouldn't be calling you. I am asking for help: Challenges influencing immigrant and refugee women's mental health. Issues in Mental Health Nursing, *32*(5), 279–90. https://doi.org/10.3109/01612840.2010.550383. Medline:21574842

Dougherty, D.D., Brennan, B.P., Stewart, S.E., Wilhelm, S., Widge, A.S., & Rauch, S.L. (2018). Neuroscientifically informed formulation and treatment planning for patients with obsessive-compulsive disorder: A review. *JAMA Psychiatry, 75*(10), 1081–7. https://doi.org/10.1001/jamapsychiatry.2013.914. Medline:30140845

Douglass, H.M., Moffitt, T.E., Dar, R., McGee, R., & Silva, P. (1995). Obsessive-compulsive disorder in a birth cohort of 18-year-olds: Prevalence and predictors. *Journal of the American Academy of Child & Adolescent Psychiatry, 34*(11), 1424–31. https://doi.org/10.1097/00004583-199511000-00008. Medline:8543509

Dowell, K.A., & Ogles, B.M. (2010). The effects of parent participation on child psychotherapy outcome: A meta-analytic review. *Journal of Clinical Child & Adolescent Psychology, 39*(2), 151–62. https://doi.org/10.1080/15374410903532585. Medline:20390807

Duncan, L., Georgiades, K., Reid, G.J., Comeau, J., Birch, S., Wang, L., & Boyle, M.H. (2020). Area-level variation in children's unmet need for community-based mental health services: Findings from the 2014 Ontario Child Health Study. *Administration and Policy in Mental Health, 15*(3), 7. https://doi.org/10.1007/s10488-020-01016-3. Medline:31974741

Du Paula, A., & Rabbitskin, N. (2018). Working with indigenous leadership and indigenous environment. In J. Wagner (Ed.), *Leadership and influencing change in nursing* (pp. 52–72). UR Press. https://leadershipandinfluencingchangeinnursing

.pressbooks.com/chapter/chapter-3-working-with-indigenous-leadership
-and-indigenous-environments/

Dyck, R., Osgood, N., Lin, T.H., Gao, A., & Stang, M.R. (2010). Epidemiology of diabetes mellitus among First Nations and non-First Nations adults. *Canadian Medical Association Journal, 182*(3), 249–56. https://doi.org/10.1503/cmaj .090846. Medline:20083562

Edge, S., Newbold, B., & McKeary, M. (2014). Exploring socio-cultural factors that mediate, facilitate, & constrain the health and empowerment of refugee youth. *Social Science & Medicine, 117*, 34–41. https://doi.org/10.1016/j .socscimed.2014.07.025. Medline:25036014

Eisen, J.L., Mancebo, M.A., Pinto, A., Coles, M.E., Pagano, M.E., Stout, R., & Rasmussen, S.A. (2006). Impact of obsessive-compulsive disorder on quality of life. *Comprehensive Psychiatry, 47*(4), 270–5. https://doi.org/10.1016/ j.comppsych.2005.11.006. Medline:16769301

Eley, T.C., Bolton, D., O'Connor, T.G., Perrin, S., Smith, P., & Plomin, R. (2003). A twin study of anxiety-related behaviours in pre-school children. *Journal of Child Psychology & Psychiatry, 44*(7), 945–60. https://doi.org /10.1111/1469-7610.00179. Medline:14531577

Ellis, B.H., Kia-Keating, M., Yusuf, S.A., Lincoln, A., Nur, A. (2007). Ethical research in refugee communities and the use of community participatory methods. *Transcult Psychiatry, 44*(3), 459–81. https://doi.org/10.1177 /1363461507081642. Medline:17938156

Elman, A., Etter, M., Fairman, K., & Chatwood, S. (2019). Mental health services in the Northwest Territories: A scoping review. *International Journal of Circumpolar Health, 78*(1), 1629783. https://doi.org/10.1080/22423982 .2019.1629783. Medline:31219779

Elsayed, D., Song, J.-H., Myatt, E., Colasante, T., & Malti, T. (2019). Anger and sadness regulation in refugee children: The roles of pre- and post-migratory factors. *Child Psychiatry & Human Development, 50*(5), 846–55. https://doi .org/10.1007/s10578-019-00887-4. Medline:30937680

Employment & Social Development Canada. (2018). *Social isolation of seniors – Supplement to the social isolation and social innovation toolkit: A focus on new immigrant and refugee seniors in Canada.* Government of Canada. www.canada .ca/en/employment-social-development/corporate/seniors/forum/social -isolation-immigrant-refugee.html

Ermine, W. (2007). The ethical space of engagement. *Indigenous Law Journal, 6*(1), 193–203.

Evans, G.W., Saltzman, H., & Cooperman, J.L. (2001). Housing quality and children's socioemotional health. *Environment & Behavior, 33*(3), 389–99. https://doi.org/10.1177/00139160121973043

Evans-Lacko, S., Aguilar-Gaxiola, S., Al-Hamzawi, A., Alonso, J., Benjet, C., Bruffaerts, R., Chiu, W.T., ... Thornicroft, G. (2018). Socio-economic variations in the mental health treatment gap for people with anxiety, mood, and substance use disorders: Results from the WHO World Mental Health (WMH) surveys. *Psychological Medicine*, *48*(9), 1560–71. https://doi.org /10.1017/S0033291717003336. Medline:29173244

Farah, M.J., Shera, D.M., Savage, J.H., Betancourt, L., Giannetta, J.M., Brodsky, N.L., ... Hurt, H. (2006). Childhood poverty: Specific associations with neurocognitive development. *Brain Research*, *1110*(1), 166–74. https://doi .org/10.1016/j.brainres.2006.06.072. Medline:16879809

Farmer, C., Thienemann, M., Leibold, C., Kamalani, G., Sauls, B., & Frankovich, J. (2018). Psychometric evaluation of the caregiver burden inventory in children and adolescents with PANS. *Journal of Pediatric Psychology*, *43*(7), 749–57. https://doi.org/10.1093/jpepsy/jsy014. Medline:29547961

Fayed, S. T., King, A., King, M., Macklin, C., Demeria, J., Rabbitskin, N., Healy, B. & Gonzales (Sempulyan), S. (2018). In the eyes of Indigenous people in Canada: Exposing the underlying colonial etiology of hepatitis C and the imperative for trauma-informed care. *Canadian Liver Journal*, *1*(3), 1–15. https://doi.org/10.3138/canlivj.2018-0009

Fazel, M., & Stein, A. (2002). The mental health of refugee children. *Archive Disease Childhood*, *87*(5), 366–70. https://doi.org/10.1136/adc.87.5.366

Fearon, G. & Wald, S. (2011). The earnings gap between black and white workers in Canada: Evidence from the 2006 Census. *Industrial Relations*, *66*(3), 321–488. https://doi.org/10.7202/1006342ar

Fenta, H., Hyman, I., & Noh, S. (2004). Determinants of depression among Ethiopian immigrants and refugees in Toronto. *The Journal of Nervous & Mental Disease*, *192*(5), 363–72. https://doi.org/10.1097/01.nmd .0000126729.08179.07. Medline:15126891

Fenta, H., Hyman, I., & Noh, S. (2006). Mental health service utilization by Ethiopian immigrants and refugees in Toronto. *The Journal of Nervous & Mental Disease*, *194*(12), 925–34. https://doi.org/10.1097/01.nmd .0000249109.71776.58. Medline:17164631

Fenta, H., Hyman, I., & Noh, S. (2007). Health service utilization by Ethiopian immigrants and refugees in Toronto. *Journal of Immigrant & Minority Health*, *9*(4), 349–57. https://doi.org/10.1007/s10903-007-9043-0. Medline:17380388

Fenton, N., Elliott, S., Vine, M., Hampson, C., Latycheva, O., Barker, K., & Gillepsie, J-A. (2012). Assessing needs: Asthma in First Nations and Inuit communities in Canada. *Pimatisiwin: A Journal of Aboriginal and Indigenous Community Health*, *10*(1), 71–81. https://www.pimatisiwin.com/online /wp-content/uploads/2012/07/06FentonElliottNew.pdf

Fernández de la Cruz, L., Kolvenbach, S., Vidal-Ribas, P., Jassi, A., Llorens, M., Patel, N., ... Mataix-Cols, D. (2016). Illness perception, help-seeking attitudes, and knowledge related to obsessive-compulsive disorder across different ethnic groups: a community survey. *Social Psychiatry & Psychiatric Epidemiology, 51*(3), 455–64. https://doi.org/10.1007/s00127-015-1144-9. Medline:26498926

Fineberg, N.A., Dell'Osso, B., Albert, U., Maina, G., Geller, D., Carmi, L., ... Zohar, J. (2019). Early intervention for obsessive compulsive disorder: An expert consensus statement. *European Neuropsychopharmacology, 29*(4), 549–65. https://doi.org/10.1016/j.euroneuro.2019.02.002. Medline:30773387

First Nations Information Governance Centre (FNIGC). (2011). *First Nations Regional Longitudinal Health Survey. RHS Phase 2 (2008/10): Preliminary results.* http://fnigc.ca/sites/default/files/RHSPreliminaryReport.pdf

First Nations Information Governance Centre (FNIGC). (2012). *First Nations Regional Health Survey (RHS) 2008/10: National report on adults, youth and children living in First Nations communities.* http://fnigc.ca/sites/default /files/docs/first_nations_regional_health_survey_rhs_2008-10_-_national _report.pdf

Flament, M.F., Whitaker, A., Rapoport, J.L., Davies, M., Berg, C.Z., Kalikow, K., Sceery, W., & Shaffer, D. (1988). Obsessive compulsive disorder in adolescence: An epidemiological study. *Journal of the American Academy of Child & Adolescent Psychiatry, 27*(6), 764–71. https://doi.org/10.1097 /00004583-198811000-00018. Medline:3264280

Fogel, J. (2003). An epidemiological perspective of obsessive-compulsive disorder in children and adolescents. *Canadian Child & Adolescent Psychiatry Review, 12*(2), 33–6. Medline:19030478

Foo, S.Q. Wilson, W.T., Ho, C.S., Tran, B.X., Nguyen, L.H., McIntyre, R.S., & Ho, R.C. (2018). Prevalence of depression among migrants: A systematic review and meta-analysis. *International Journal of Environmental Research and Public Health, 15*(9), 1986. https://doi.org/10.3390/ijerph15091986. Medline:30213071

Francis, J. (2009). *"Hanging on the edge of the house" – Poor housing outcomes and risk of homelessness among African refugees.* https://open.library.ubc.ca/cIRcle /collections/ubctheses/24/items/1.0068565

Francis, J. (2010). Poor housing outcomes among African refugees in metro Vancouver. *Canadian Issues,* (Fall), 59–62.

Freeman, J.B., Benito, K., Herren, J., Kemp, J., Sung, J., Georgiadis, C., Arora, A., Walther, M., & Garcia, A. (2018). Evidence base update of psychosocial treatments for pediatric obsessive-compulsive disorder: Evaluating, improving, and transporting what works. *Journal of Clinical Child & Adolescent Psychology, 47*(5), 669–98. https://doi.org/10.1080/15374416.2018.1496443. Medline:30130414

Freeman, J.B., Garcia, A.M., Coyne, L., Ale, C., Przeworski, A., Himle, M., Compton, S., & Leonard, H.L. (2008). Early childhood OCD: Preliminary findings from a family-based cognitive-behavioral approach. *Journal of the*

American Academy of Child & Adolescent Psychiatry, 47(5), 593–602. https://doi
.org/10.1097/CHI.0b013e31816765f9. Medline:18356758

Galabuzi, G.E. (2005). *Canada's economic apartheid: The social exclusion of racialized
groups in the new century.* Canadian Scholars' Press.

Garcia, A.M., Sapyta, J.J., Moore, P.S., Freeman, J.B., Franklin, M.E., March,
J.S., & Foa, E.B. (2010). Predictors and moderators of treatment outcome in
the Pediatric Obsessive Compulsive Treatment Study (POTS I). *Journal of the
American Academy of Child & Adolescent Psychiatry, 49*(10), 1024–33. https://
doi.org/10.1016/j.jaac.2010.06.013. Medline:20855047

García-Soriano, G., Rufer, M., Delsignore, A., & Weidt, S. (2014). Factors
associated with non-treatment or delayed treatment seeking in OCD
sufferers: A review of the literature. *Psychiatry Research, 220*(1–2), 1–10.
https://doi.org/10.1016/j.psychres.2014.07.009. Medline:25108591

Garwick, A.W., & Seppelt, A.M. (2010). Developing a family-centered
participatory action project. *Journal of Family Nursing, 16*(3), 269–81. https://
doi.org/10.1177/1074840710376175. Medline:20686103

Gatov, E., Muir, L., Mowat, V., Elkader, A., Yang, J., Kopp, A., & Cairney,
J. (2020). Acute and outpatient service utilisation prior to, during, and
following enrolment in community-based mental health treatment among
children and youth in Central Ontario: A proof of concept for cross-sectoral
data linkage. *Journal of Paediatric Child Health, 11*, 7. https://doi.org/10.1111
/jpc.14779. Medline:31997491

Geller, D. A., Abramovitch, A., Mittelman, A., Stark, A., Ramsey, K.,
Cooperman, A., Baer, L., & Stewart, S. E. (2018). Neurocognitive function
in paediatric obsessive-compulsive disorder. *World Journal of Biological
Psychiatry, 19*(2), 142–51. https://doi.org/10.1080/15622975.2017.1282173.
Medline:28090807

Geller, D.A., Biederman, J., Faraone, S.V., Frazier, J., Coffey, B J., Kim, G., &
Bellordre, C.A. (2000). Clinical correlates of obsessive compulsive disorder in
children and adolescents referred to specialized and non-specialized clinical
settings. *Depression and Anxiety, 11*(4), 163–8. https://doi.org/10.1002/1520
-6394. Medline:10945136

Geller, D.A., Biederman, J., Jones, J., Park, K., Schwartz, S., Shapiro, S., &
Coffey, B. (1998). Is juvenile obsessive-compulsive disorder a developmental
subtype of the disorder? A review of the pediatric literature. *Journal of the
American Academy of Child & Adolescent Psychiatry, 37*(4), 420–7. https://doi
.org/10.1097/00004583-199804000-00020. Medline:9549963

Geller, D.A., & March, J.S. (2012). Practice parameter for the assessment and
treatment of children and adolescents with obsessive-compulsive disorder
[for the AACAP Committee on Quality Issues]. *Journal of the American Academy
of Child & Adolescent Psychiatry, 51*(1), 98–113. https://doi.org/10.1016/j
.jaac.2011.09.019

Georgiades, K., Duncan, L., Wang, L., Comeau, J., Boyle, M.H., & Ontario Child Health Study Team. (2019). Six-month prevalence of mental disorders and service contacts among children and youth in Ontario: Evidence from the 2014 Ontario Child Health Study. *Canadian Journal of Psychiatry, 64*(4), 246–55. https://doi.org/10.1177/0706743719830024. Medline:30978138

Georgiades, K., Paksarian, D., Rudolph, K.E., & Merikangas, K.R. (2018). Prevalence of mental disorder and service use by immigrant generation and race/ethnicity among U.S. adolescents. *Journal of the American Academy of Child & Adolescent Psychiatry, 57*(4), 280–7.e282. https://doi.org/10.1016/j.jaac.2018.01.020. Medline:29588054

Gessner, B.D., & Neeno T. (2005). Trends in asthma prevalence, hospitalization risk, and inhaled corticosteroid use among Alaska Native and non-native Medicaid recipients younger than 20 years. *Annals of Allergy, Asthma & Immunology, 94*(3), 372–9. https://doi.org/10.1016/S1081-1206(10)60990-8

Gionet, L. & Roshanafshar, S. (2015). Select health indicators of First Nations people living off reserve, Métis and Inuit. Statistics Canada, Cat. no. 82-624-x. https://www150.statcan.gc.ca/n1/pub/82-624-x/2013001/article/11763-eng.htm

Gladden, J. (2012). The coping skills of East African refugees: A literature review. *Refugee Survey Quarterly, 31*(3), 177–96. https://doi.org/10.1093/rsq/hds009

Global Initiative for Asthma (GINA). (2020). *Global strategy for asthma management and prevention (2020 update).* www.ginasthma.org

Goodman, A., Fleming, K., Markwick, N., Morrison, T., Lagimodiere, L., & Kerr, T. (2017). "They treated me like crap and I know it was because I was native": The healthcare experiences of Aboriginal peoples living in Vancouver's inner city. *Social Science & Medicine, 178*, 87–94. https://doi.org/10.1016/j.socscimed.2017.01.053. Medline:28214449

Goodwin, R., Koenen, K.C., Hellman, F., Guardino, M., & Struening, E. (2002). Helpseeking and access to mental health treatment for obsessive-compulsive disorder. *Acta Psychiatrica Scandinavica, 106*(2), 143–9. https://doi.org/10.1034/j.1600-0447.2002.01221.x. Medline:12121213

Gottlieb, B.H. (2000). Accomplishments and challenges in social support intervention research. In M. Stewart (Ed.), *Chronic conditions and caregiving in Canada: Social support strategies* (pp. 294–310). University of Toronto Press.

Gottlieb, B.H., & Bergen, A.E. (2010). Social support concepts and measures. *Journal of Psychsomatic Research, 69*(5), 511–20. https://doi.org/10.1016j.jpsychores.2009.10.001. Medline:20955871

Government of British Columbia. (2020). *In plain sight: Addressing Indigenous-specific racism and discrimination in B.C. health care.* https://engage.gov.bc.ca/app/uploads/sites/613/2020/11/In-Plain-Sight-Full-Report.pdf

Government of Canada. (2013). What makes Canadians healthy or unhealthy? www.canada.ca/en/public-health/services/health-promotion/population -health/what-determines-health/what-makes-canadians-healthy-unhealthy.html

Government of Canada. (2014). Research involving the First Nations, Inuit, and Metis Peoples of Canada. In Council Policy Statement: Ethical Conduct for Research Involving Humans (chap. 9). www.pre.ethics.gc.ca/eng/policy -politique/initiatives/tcps2-eptc2/Default/

Government of Canada. (2015). *Rio political declaration on social determinants of health: A snapshot of Canadian actions 2015.* www.canada.ca/en/public-health /services/publications/science-research-data/rio-political-declaration-social -determinants-health-snapshot-canadian-actions-2015.html

Government of Canada. (2018a). *Social determinants of health and health inequities.* www.canada.ca/en/public-health/services/health-promotion /population-health/what-determines-health.html

Government of Canada. (2018b). *Key health inequalities in Canada: A national portrait – executive summary.* www.canada.ca/en/public-health/services /publications/science-research-data/key-health-inequalities-canada-national -portrait-executive-summary.html

Government of Canada. (2018c). *Canada: A history of refuge.* https://www .canada.ca/en/immigration-refugees-citizenship/services/refugees/history .html

Government of Canada. (2018d). *Syrian refugees – Monthly IRCC updates.* https://open.canada.ca/data/en/dataset/01c85d28-2a81-4295-9c06 -4af792a7c209

Government of Canada. (2018e). *Prescription drug insurance coverage.* www.canada.ca/en/health-canada/services/health-care-system /pharmaceuticals/access-insurance-coverage-prescription-medicines.html

Government of Canada. (2019). *Understanding the report on key health inequities in Canada.* www.canada.ca/en/public-health/services/publications /science-research-data/understanding-report-key-health-inequalities -canada.html

Grace, S.L., Tan, Y., Cribbie, R.A., Nguyen, H., Ritvo, P., & Irvine, J. (2016). The mental health status of ethnocultural minorities in Ontario and their mental health care. *BMC Psychiatry, 16*(1), 47. https://doi.org/10.1186/s12888-016 -0759-z. Medline:26915910

Gracey, M., & King, M. (2009). Indigenous health part 1: Determinants and disease patterns. *Lancet, 374*(9683), 65–75. https://doi.org/10.1016/S0140 -6736(09)60914-4. Medline:19577695

Grandner, M.A., Jackson, N.J., Izci-Balserak, B., Gallagher, R.A., Murray-Bachmann, R., Williams, N.J., ... Jean-Louis, G. (2015). Social and behavioral determinants of perceived insufficient sleep. *Frontiers in Neurology, 6,* 112. https://doi.org/10.3389/fneur.2015.00112. Medline:26097464

Greenglass, E.R., Schwarzer, R., & Taubert, S. (1999). *The Proactive Coping Inventory (PCI): A multidimensional research instrument.* York University. http://userpage.fu-berlin.de/~health/greenpci.htm

Greenwood, M.L., & de Leeuw, S.N. (2012). Social determinants of health and the future well-being of Aboriginal children in Canada. *Paediatric Child Health, 17*(7), 381–4. https://doi.org/10.1093/pch/17.7.381. Medline:23904782

Grewal, S.K., Bhagat, R., & Balneaves, L.G. (2008). Perinatal beliefs and practices of immigrant Punjabi women living in Canada. *Journal of Obstetric, Gynecologic & Neonatal Nursing, 37*(3), 290–300. https://doi.org/10.1111/j.1552-6909.2008.00234.x. Medline:18507600

Grover, S., & Dutt, A. (2011). Perceived burden and quality of life of caregivers in obsessive-compulsive disorder. *Psychiatry & Clinical Neurosciences, 65*(5), 416–22. https://doi.org/10.1111/j.1440-1819.2011.02240.x. Medline:21851450

Grover, S., Patra, B.N., Aggarwal, M., Avasthi, A., Chakrabarti, S., & Malhotra, S. (2014). Relationship of supernatural beliefs and first treatment contact in patients with obsessive compulsive disorder: An exploratory study from India. *International Journal of Social Psychiatry, 60*(8), 818–27. https://doi.org/10.1177/0020764014527266. Medline:24663395

Gruzd, A., Staves, K., & Wilk, A. (2012). Connected scholars: Examining the role of social media in research practices of faculty using the UTAUT model. *Computers in Human Behavior, 28*(6), 2340–50. https://doi.org/10.1016/j.chb.2012.07.004

Guèvremont, A., Carrière, G., Bougie, E., & Kohen, D. (2017). Health reports: Acute care hospitalization of Aboriginal children and youth. Statistics Canada, Cat. no. 82-003-x. https://www150.statcan.gc.ca/n1/pub/82-003-x/2017007/article/14844-eng.htm

Guruge, S., & Butt, H. (2015). A scoping review of mental health issues and concerns among immigrant and refugee youth in Canada: Looking back, moving forward. *Canadian Journal of Public Health, 106*(2), e72–8. https://doi.org/10.17269/CJPH.106.4588. Medline:25955675

Hadfield, K., Ostrowski, A., & Ungar, M. (2017). What can we expect of the mental health and well-being of Syrian refugee children and adolescents in Canada? *Canadian Psychology, 58*(2), 194–201. https://doi.org/10.1037/cap0000102

Hale, D.R., & Viner, R.M. (2018). How adolescent health influences education and employment: Investigating longitudinal associations and mechanisms. *Journal of Epidemiology & Community Health, 72*(6), 465–70. https://doi.org/10.1136/jech-2017-209605. Medline:29615474

Hall-Lande, J.A., Eisenberg, M.E., Christenson, S.L., & Neumark-Sztainer, D. (2007). Social isolation, psychological health, and protective factors in adolescence. *Adolescence, 42*(166), 265–85. Medline:17849936

Halseth, R., & Greenwood, M. (2019). *Indigenous early childhood development in Canada: Current state of knowledge and future directions.*National Collaborating Centre for Aboriginal Health. https://www.nccah-ccnsa.ca/docs/health/RPT-ECD-PHAC-Greenwood-Halseth-EN.pdf

Halseth, R. & Murdock, L. (2020). *Supporting Indigenous self-determination in health: Lessons learned from a review of best practices in health governance in Canada and internationally.* National Collaborating Centre for Aboriginal Health. https://nccih.ca/Publications/Lists/Publications/Attachments/317/Ind-Self-Determine-Halseth-Murdoch-EN-web-2020-12-02.pdf

Hamdullahpur, K., Jacobs, K.W.J., & Gill, K.J. (2017). A comparison of socioeconomic status and mental health among inner-city Aboriginal and non-Aboriginal women. *International Journal of Circumpolar Health, 76*(1), 1340693. https://doi.org/10.1080/22423982.2017.1340693. Medline:28747094

Hanson, E. (2009). *Sixties Scoop:* The Sixties Scoop & Aboriginal child welfare. https://indigenousfoundations.arts.ubc.ca/sixties_scoop/

Hansson, E.K., Tuck, A., Lurie, S., & McKenzie, K. (2012). Rates of mental illness and suicidality in immigrant, refugee, ethnocultural, and racialized groups in Canada: A review of the literature. *Canadian Journal of Psychiatry, 57*(2), 111–21. https://doi.org/10.1177/070674371205700208. Medline:22340151

Harder, H.G., Rash, J., Holyk, T., Jovel, E., & Harder, K. (2012). Indigenous youth suicide: A systematic review of the literature. *Pimatisiwin: A Journal of Aboriginal and Indigenous Community Health, 10*(1), 126–42.

Hassan, G., & Rousseau, C. (2009). North African and Latin American parents' and adolescents' perceptions of physical discipline and physical abuse: when dysnormativity begets exclusion. *Child Welfare, 88*(6), 5–23. Medline:20695289

Hawthorne, G. (2006). Measuring social isolation in older adults: Development and initial validation of the friendship scale. *Social Indicators Research, 77*(3), 521–48. https://doi.org/10.1007/s11205-005-7746-y

Health Canada. (2019). *Social determinants of health and health inequalities.* https://www.canada.ca/en/public-health/services/health-promotion/population-health/what-determines-health.html

Henderson, J.L., Chaim, G., Hawke, L.D., & National Youth Screening Project Network (2017). Screening for substance use and mental health problems in a cross-sectoral sample of Canadian youth. *International Journal of Mental Health Systems, 11*(1), 21. https://doi.org/10.1186/s13033-017-0128-4. Medline:28261324

Herring, S., Gray, K., Taffe, J., Tonge, B., Sweeney, D., & Einfeld, S. (2006). Behaviour and emotional problems in toddlers with pervasive developmental disorders and developmental delay: Associations with parental mental health and family functioning. *Journal of Intellectual Disability Research, 50*(12), 874–82. https://doi.org/10.1111/j.1365-2788.2006.00904.x. Medline:17100948

Heyman, I., Fombonne, E., Simmons, H., Ford, T., Meltzer, H., & Goodman, R. (2001). Prevalence of obsessive-compulsive disorder in the British nationwide survey of child mental health. *British Journal of Psychiatry, 179*, 324–9. https://doi.org/10.1192/bjp.179.4.324. Medline:11581112

Hibbs, E.D., Hamburger, S.D., Kruesi, M.J., & Lenane, M. (1993). Factors affecting expressed emotion in parents of ill and normal children. *American Journal of Orthopsychiatry, 63*(1), 103–12. https://doi.org/10.1037/h0079395. Medline:8427300

Hilario, C.T., Oliffe, J.L., Wong, J.P.H., Browne, A.J., & Johnson, J.L. (2015). Migration and young people's mental health in Canada: A scoping review. *Journal of Mental Health, 24*(6), 414–22. https://doi.org/10.3109/09638237.2015.1078881. Medline:26556308

Hilario, C.T., Vo, D.X., Johnson, J.L., & Saewyc, E.M. (2014). Acculturation, gender, and mental health of Southeast Asian immigrant youth in Canada. *Journal of Immigrant and Minority Health, 16*(6), 1121–9. https://doi.org/10.1007/s10903-014-9978-x. Medline:24469590

Hilario, C.T., Vo, D.X., & Pottie, K. (2015). *Immigrant adolescent health: Background and context. Caring for kids new to Canada.* Canadian Pediatric Society. www.kidsnewtocanada.ca/culture/adolescent-health-background

Himle, J.A., Muroff, J.R., Taylor, R.J., Baser, R.E., Abelson, J.M., Hanna, G.L., Abelson, J.L., & Jackson, J.S. (2008). Obsessive-compulsive disorder among African Americans and blacks of Caribbean descent: Results from the National Survey of American Life. *Depression and Anxiety, 25*(12), 993–1005. https://doi.org/10.1002/da.20434. Medline:18833577

Hodes, M., & Vostanis, P. (2019). Practitioner review: Mental health problems of refugee children and adolescents and their management. *Journal of Child Psychology and Psychiatry, 60*(7), 716–31. Medline:30548855

Horwath, E., & Weissman, M.M. (2000). The epidemiology and cross-national presentation of obsessive-compulsive disorder. *Psychiatric Clinics of North America, 23*(3), 493–507. https://doi.org/10.1016/S0193-953X(05)70176-3. Medline:10986723

Hou, F., Schellenberg, G., & Berry, J. (2016). Patterns and determinants of immigrants' sense of belonging to Canada and their source country. Statistics Canada, Cat. no. 11F0019M-no. 383. https://www150.statcan.gc.ca/n1/pub/11f0019m/11f0019m2016383-eng.htm

Houtepen, L.C., Heron, J., Suderman, M.J., Fraser, A., Chittleborough, C.R., & Howe, L.D. (2020). Associations of adverse childhood experiences with educational attainment and adolescent health and the role of family and socioeconomic factors: A prospective cohort study in the UK. *PLoS*

Medicine, 17(3), e1003031. https://doi.org/10.1371/journal.pmed.1003031. Medline:32119668

Indigenous Services Canada. (2018). *Improving child and family services in Indigenous communities: Survey of summary report.* Government of Canada. https://www.sac-isc.gc.ca/eng/1530823640599/1535381807721

Inozu, M., Karanci, A.N., & Clark, D.A. (2012). Why are religious individuals more obsessional? The role of mental control beliefs and guilt in Muslims and Christians. *Journal of Behavior Therapy & Experimental Psychiatry, 43*(3), 959–66. https://doi.org/10.1016/j.jbtep.2012.02.004. Medline:22484698

Institute for Integrative Science & Health. (2018). *Two-Eyed seeing.* Cape Breton University. http://www.integrativescience.ca/Principles/TwoEyedSeeing/

Institute of Fiscal Studies and Democracy (IFSD). (2020). *Funding First Nations child and family services (FNCFS): A performance budget approach to well-being.* University of Ottawa. https://www.afn.ca/wp-content /uploads/2020/09/2020-09-09_Final-report_Funding-First-Nations-child -and-family-services.pdf

International Organization for Migration. (2018). *World migration report (2018).* International Organization for Migration. https://publications.iom.int /system/files/pdf/wmr_2018_en.pdf

Islam, F. (2015). Immigrating to Canada during early childhood associated with increased risk for mood disorders. *Community Mental Health Journal, 51*(6), 723–32. https://doi.org/10.1007/s10597-015-9851-y. Medline:25725782

Islam, F., Khanlou, N., & Tamim, H. (2014). South Asian populations in Canada: Migration and mental health. *BMC Psychiatry, 14*(1), 154. https:// doi.org/10.1186/1471-244X-14-154. Medline:24884792

Ismaila, A.S., Sayani, A.P., Marin, M., & Su, Z. (2013). Clinical, economic, and humanistic burden of asthma in Canada: A systematic review. *BMC Pulmonary Medicine, 13*, 70. https://doi.org/10.1186/1471-2466-13-70. Medline:24304726

Ivarsson, T., Skarphedinsson, G., Kornor, H., Axelsdottir, B., Biedilae, S., Heyman, I., ... Accreditation Task Force of the Canadian Institute for Obsessive Compulsive Disorder. (2015). The place of and evidence for serotonin reuptake inhibitors (SRIs) for obsessive compulsive disorder (OCD) in children and adolescents: Views based on a systematic review and meta-analysis. *Psychiatry Research, 227*(1), 93–103. https://doi.org /10.1016/j.psychres.2015.01.015. Medline:25769521

Jack, E.M., Chartier, M.J., Ly, G., Fortier, J., Murdock, N., Cochrane, B., ... Sareen, J. (2020). School personnel and community members' perspectives in implementing PAX good behaviour game in first nations grade 1 classrooms. *International Journal of Circumpolar Health, 79*(1), 1735052. https://doi.org/10.1080/22423982.2020.1735052. Medline:32102633

Jafari, F. (2017). *Strengths-based therapy*. Nashre Elm.

Jakovljevic, I., Miller, A.P., & Fitzgerald, B. (2016). Children's mental health: Is poverty the diagnosis? *BC Medical Journal, 58*(8), 454–60.

Jaranson, J., Butcher, J., Halcon, L. Johnson, D.R., Robertson, C., Savik, K., ... Westermeyer, J. (2004). Somali and Oromo refugees: Correlates of torture and trauma history. *American Journal of Public Health, 94*(4), 591–8. https://doi.org/10.2105/AJPH.94.4.591. Medline:15054011

Jaspers-Fayer, F., Lin, S.Y., Belschner, L., Mah, J., Chan, E., Bleakley, C., ... Stewart, S.E. (2018). A case-control study of sleep disturbances in pediatric obsessive-compulsive disorder. *Journal of Anxiety Disorders, 55*, 1–7. https://doi.org/10.1016/j.janxdis.2018.02.001. Medline:29529448

Jaspers-Fayer, F., Negreiros, J., Lin, S.Y., Belschner, L., & Stewart, S.E. (2017). Cognitive planning neural correlates in a pediatric monozygotic twin pair discordant for obsessive-compulsive disorder: Exploring potential application in precision medicine. *Journal of Clinical Psychiatry, 78*(9), e1320–e1321. https://doi.org/10.4088/JCP.16cr10967. Medline:29345872

Jetty, R. (2017). Tobacco use and misuse among Indigenous children and youth in Canada. *Pediatric Child Health, 22*(7), 395–9. https://doi.org/10.1093/pch/pxx124. Medline:29491724

Jones, S. (1998). *The archaeology of ethnicity: Constructing identities in the past and present*. Routledge.

Kalra, S.K., & Swedo, S.E. (2009). Children with obsessive-compulsive disorder: Are they just "little adults"? *Journal of Clinical Investigation, 119*(4), 737–46. https://doi.org/10.1172/JCI37563. Medline:19339765

Karno, M., Golding, J.M., Sorenson, S.B., & Burnam, M.A. (1988). The epidemiology of obsessive-compulsive disorder in five US communities. *Archives of General Psychiatry, 45*(12), 1094–9. https://doi.org/10.1001/archpsyc.1988.01800360042006. Medline:3264144

Karunanayake, C.P., Amin, K., Abonyi, S., Dosman, J.A., & Pahwa, P. (2019). Prevalence and determinants of asthma among aboriginal adolescents in Canada. *Journal of Asthma, 57*(1), 40–6. https://doi.org/10.1080/02770903.2018.1541354. Medline:30628527

Keller, B., Labrique, A., Jain, K.M., Pekosz, A., & Levine, O. (2014). Mind the gap: Social media engagement by public health researchers. *Journal of Medical Internet Research, 16*(1), e8. https://doi.org/10.2196/jmir.2982. Medline:24425670

Kelly, M. (2011). Toward a new era of policy: Health care service delivery to First Nations. *International Indigenous Policy Journal, 2*(1), 11. https://ezproxy.tru.ca/login?url=https://search.ebscohost.com/login.aspx?direct=true&db=edsdoj&AN=edsdoj.0f8ed3d1c5464bada6feb653c3523556&site=eds-live

Kenney, M.K., & Chanlongbutra, A. (2020). Prevalence of parent reported health conditions among 0- to 17-year-olds in rural United States: National Survey of Children's Health, 2016–2017. *Journal of Rural Health, 15*(3), 3278. https://doi.org/10.1111/jrh.12411. Medline:32045063

Kenny, C. (2012). Liberating leadership theory. In C. Kenny & T. Ngaroimata Fraser (Eds.), *Living Indigenous leadership: Native narratives on building strong communities* (pp. 1–16). UBC Press.

Khan, E. (2019). Mental health challenges and interventions for refugee children. American Psychological Association, 23 July. https://www.apa .org/international/global-insights/refugee-children-challenges

Kidd, S.A., Thistle, J., Beaulieu, T., O'Grady, B., & Gaetz, S. (2019). A national study of Indigenous youth homelessness in Canada. *Public Health, 176,* 163–71. https://doi.org/10.1016/j.puhe.2018.06.012. Medline:30143269

Kim, K.L., Christensen, R.E., Ruggieri, A., Schettini, E., Freeman, J.B., Garcia, A.M., … Dickstein, D.P. (2019). Cognitive performance of youth with primary generalized anxiety disorder versus primary obsessive-compulsive disorder. *Depression and Anxiety, 36*(2), 130–40. https://doi.org/10.1002/da.22848. Medline:30375085

King, M. (2010). Chronic diseases and mortality in Canadian Aboriginal peoples: Learning from the knowledge. Chronic Diseases in Canada, *31*(1), 2–3. Medline:21176410

King, M., Zayas, G., & Martial, R. (2004). Cardiovascular and respiratory health risks in Canada's Aboriginal population. *Pimatisiwin: A Journal of Aboriginal and Indigenous Community Health,* 2(2): 75–95. https:// journalindigenouswellbeing.com/media/2018/10/5_King.pdf

Kinghorn, B., Fretts, A.M., O'Leary, R.A., Karr, C.J., Rosenfeld, M., & Best, L.G. (2019). Socioeconomic and environmental risk factors for pediatric asthma in an American Indian community. *Academic Pediatrics, 19*(6), 631–7. https:// doi.org/10.1016/j.acap.2019.05.006. Medline:31103883

Kirmayer, L., Narasiah, L., Munoz, M., Rashid, M., Ryder, A.G. … Pottie, K. (2011). Common mental health problems in immigrants and refugees: General approach in primary care. *Canadian Medical Association Journal, 183*(12), E959–67. https://doi.org/10.1503/cmaj.090292. Medline:20603342

Kisely, S., Terashima, M., & Langille, D. (2008). A population-based analysis of the health experience of African Nova Scotians. *Canadian Medical Association Journal, 179*(7), 653–58. https://doi.org/10.1503/cmaj.071279. Medline:18809896

Kohen, D.E., Bougie, E., & Guèvremont, A. (2015). Housing and health among Inuit children. *Health Reports,* 26(11), 21–7. Medline:26583694

Kon, A., Lou, E., MacDonald, M.A., Riak, A., & Smarsh, L. (2012). *Working with South Sudanese immigrant students – teacher resources.* Canadian Multicultural Education Foundation and Alberta Teachers Association. www.teachers.ab.ca

/SiteCollectionDocuments/ATA/For%20Members/ProfessionalDevelopment
/Diversity-Equity-and-Human-Rights/AR-CMEF-2.pdf

Kopel, L.S., Phipatanakul, W., & Gaffin, J.M. (2014). Social disadvantage and asthma control in children. *Paediatric Respiratory Review*, *15*, 256–62. https://doi.org/10.1016/j.prrv.2014.04.017. Medline:24928775

Koran, L.M., Thienemann, M.L., & Davenport, R. (1996). Quality of life for patients with obsessive-compulsive disorder. *American Journal of Psychiatry*, *153*(6), 783–8. https://doi.org/10.1176/ajp.153.6.783

Kovesi, T. (2012). Respiratory disease in Canadian First Nations and Inuit children. *Paediatrics and Child Health*, *17*(7), 376–80. https://doi.org/10.1093/pch/17.7.376. Medline:23904781

Kozloff, N., Stergiopoulos, V., Adair, C.E., Cheung, A.H., Misir, V., Townley, G., ... Goering, P. (2016). The unique needs of homeless youths with mental illness: Baseline findings from a housing first trial. *Psychiatric Services*, *67*(10), 1083–90. https://doi.org/10.1176/appi.ps.201500461. Medline:27247178

Kurtz, D.L.M., Turner, D., Nyberg, J., & Moar, D. (2014). Social justice and health equity: Urban Aboriginal women's actions for health reform. *International Journal of Health, Wellness, and Society*, *3*(4), 13-26. https://doi.org/10.18848/2156-8960/CGP/v03i04/41081

Kwak, K. (2016). An evaluation of the healthy immigrant effect with adolescents in Canada: Examinations of gender and length of residence. *Social Science & Medicine*, *157*, 87–95. https://doi.org/10.1016/j.socscimed.2016.03.017. Medline:27064656

Kwak, K. & Rudmin, F. (2014). Adolescent health and adaptation in Canada: Examination of gender and age aspects of the healthy immigrant effect. International Journal for Equity in Health, *13*(1): 103. https://doi.org/10.1186/s12939-014-0103-5. Medline:25394371

Kyngas, H.A. (2004). Support network of adolescents with chronic disease: Adolescents' perspective. *Nursing and Health Sciences*, *6*(4), 287–93. https://doi.org/10.1111/j.1442-2018.2004.00207.x. Medline:15507049

Lambert, J. E., Holzer, J., & Hasbun, A. (2014). Association between parents' PTSD severity and children's psychological distress: A meta-analysis. *Journal of Traumatic Stress*, *27*(1), 9–17. https://doi.org/10.1002/jts.21891. Medline:24464491

Larson, B., Herx, L., Williamson, T., & Crowshoe, L. (2011). Beyond the barriers: Family medicine residents' attitudes towards providing Aboriginal health care. *Medical Education*, *45*(4), 400–6. https://doi.org/10.1111/j.1365-2923.2010.03892.x. Medline:21401688

Lavoie, J.G., Boulton, A.F., & Gervais, L. (2012). Regionalization as an opportunity for meaningful Indigenous participation in healthcare: Comparing Canada and New Zealand. *International Indigenous Policy Journal*, *3*(1), 1–14. https://doi.org/10.18584/iipj.2012.3.1.2

Lebowitz, E.R. (2017). Family impairment associated with childhood obsessive-compulsive disorder. *Journal of the American Academy of Child & Adolescent Psychiatry, 56*(3), 187–8. https://doi.org/10.1016/j.jaac.2017.01.002. Medline:28219483

Lebowitz, E.R., & Shimshoni, Y. (2018). The SPACE program, a parent-based treatment for childhood and adolescent OCD: The case of Jasmine. *Bulletin of the Menninger Clinic, 82*(4), 266–87. https://doi.org/10.1521/bumc.2018.82.4.266. Medline:30589579

Lebowitz, E.R., Vitulano, L.A., & Omer, H. (2011). Coercive and disruptive behaviors in pediatric obsessive compulsive disorder: A qualitative analysis. *Psychiatry, 74*(4), 362–71. https://doi.org/10.1521/psyc.2011.74.4.362. Medline:22168296

Leckman, J.F., King, R.A., Gilbert, D.L., Coffey, B.J., Singer, H.S., Dure, L.S.T., … Kaplan, E.L. (2011). Streptococcal upper respiratory tract infections and exacerbations of tic and obsessive-compulsive symptoms: A prospective longitudinal study. *Journal of the American Academy of Child & Adolescent Psychiatry, 50*(2), 108–18.e103. https://doi.org/10.1016/j.jaac.2010.10.011. Medline:21241948

Lemstra, M., Neudorf, C., Mackenbach, J., Darcy, C., Scott, C., Kershaw, T., & Nannapaneni, U. (2008). Risk indicators for depressed mood in youth: Limited association with Aboriginal cultural status. *Paediatr Child Health, 13*(4), 285–90. https://doi.org/10.1093/pch/13.4.285. Medline:19337594

Lenhard, F., Andersson, E., Mataix-Cols, D., Rück, C., Vigerland, S., Högström, J., … Serlachius, E. (2017). Therapist-guided, internet-delivered cognitive-behavioral therapy for adolescents with obsessive-compulsive disorder: A randomized controlled trial. *Journal of the American Academy of Child & Adolescent Psychiatry, 56*(1), 10–19.e12. https://doi.org/10.1016/j.jaac.2016.09.515. Medline:27993223

Leonard, H.L., Lenane, M.C., Swedo, S.E., Rettew, D.C., Gershon, E.S., & Rapoport, J.L. (1992). Tics and Tourette's disorder: A 2- to 7-year follow-up of 54 obsessive-compulsive children. *American Journal of Psychiatry, 149*(9), 1244–51. https://doi.org/10.1176/ajp.149.9.1244. Medline:1503140

Leonard, R.C., Franklin, M.E., Wetterneck, C.T., Riemann, B.C., Simpson, H.B., Kinnear, K., … Lake, P.M. (2016). Residential treatment outcomes for adolescents with obsessive-compulsive disorder. *Psychotherapy Research, 26*(6), 727–36. https://doi.org/10.1080/10503307.2015.1065022. Medline:26308588

Lesser, J., & Koniak-Griffin, D. (2013). Using qualitative inquiry and participatory research approaches to develop prevention research: Validating a life course perspective. *Family and Community Health, 36*(1), 34–41. https://doi.org/10.1097/FCH.0b013e31826d75a7. Medline:23168344

Letourneau, N.L., Anis, L., Ntanda, H., Novick, J., Steele, M., Steele, H., & Hart, M. (2020). Attachment & Child Health (ATTACH) pilot trials: Effect of parental reflective function intervention for families affected by toxic stress. *Infant Mental Health Journal, 41*(4), 445–62. https://doi.org/10.1002/imhj.21833. Medline:32533796

Letourneau, N. L., Duffett-Leger, L., Stewart, M., Hegadoren, K., Dennis, C., Rinaldi, C., & Stoppard, J. (2007). Canadian mothers' perceived support needs during postpartum depression. *Journal of Obstetric, Gynecologic & Neonatal Nursing, 36*(5), 441–9. https://doi.org/10.1111/j.1552-6909.2007.00174.x. Medline:17880314

Letourneau, N. L., Secco, L., Colpitts, J., Aldous, S., Stewart, M., & Dennis, C. L. (2015). Quasi-experimental evaluation of a telephone-based peer support intervention for maternal depression. *Journal of Advanced Nursing, 71*(7), 1587–99. https://doi.org/10.1111/jan.12622. Medline:25705786

Letourneau, N.L., Tryphonopoulos, P., Duffett-Leger, L., Stewart, M., Benzies, K., Dennis, C., & Joschko, J. (2012). Support intervention needs and preferences of fathers affected by postpartum depression. *Journal of Perinatal & Neonatal Nursing, 26*(1), 69–80. https://doi.org/10.1097/JPN.0b013e318241da87. Medline:22293644

Letourneau, N.L., Young, C., Secco, L., Stewart, M., Hughes, J., & Critchley, K. (2011). Supporting mothering: Service providers' perspectives of mothers and young children affected by intimate partner violence. *Research in Nursing & Health, 34*(3), 192–203. https://doi.org/10.1002/nur.20428. Medline:21391219

Lévesque, I.S., & Abdel-Baki, A. (2019). Homeless youth with first-episode psychosis: A 2-year outcome study. *Schizophrenia Research, 216*, 460–9. https://doi.org/10.1016/j.schres.2019.10.031

Lewis-Fernandez, R., Aggarwal, N.K., Baarnhielm, S., Rohlof, H., Kirmayer, L.J., Weiss, M.G., … Lu, F. (2014). Culture and psychiatric evaluation: operationalizing cultural formulation for DSM-5. *Psychiatry, 77*(2), 130–54. https://doi.org/10.1521/psyc.2014.77.2.130. Medline:24865197

Li, Y., Allen, J., & Casillas, A. (2017). Relating psychological and social factors to academic performance: A longitudinal investigation of high-poverty middle school students. *Journal of Adolescence, 56*, 179–89. https://doi.org/10.1016/j.adolescence.2017.02.007. Medline:28273555

Li, Y., Marques, L., Hinton, D.E., Wang, Y., & Xiao, Z.P. (2009). Symptom dimensions in Chinese patients with obsessive-compulsive disorder. *CNS Neuroscience & Therapeutics, 15*(3), 276–82. https://doi.org/10.1111/j.1755-5949.2009.00099.x. Medline:19691547

Lincoln, A.K., Lazarevic, V., White, M.T., & Ellis, B.H. (2016). The impact of acculturation style and acculturative hassles on the mental health of Somali adolescent refugees. *Journal of Immigrant & Minority Health, 18*(4), 771–8. https://doi.org/10.1007/s10903-015-0232-y. Medline:26048358

Linton, J.M., Green, A., & The Council on Community Pediatrics. (2019). Providing care for children in immigrant families. *Pediatrics, 144*(3), e20192077. https://doi.org/10.1542/peds.2019-2077. Medline:31427460

Lu, C., & Ng, E. (2019). Healthy immigrant effect by immigrant category in Canada. *Health Reports, 30*(4), 3–11. https://doi.org/10.25318/82-003 -x201900400001-eng. Medline:30994921

Lukemeyer, A., Meyers, M.K., & Smeeding, T. (2004). Expensive children in poor families: Out-of-pocket expenditures for the care of disabled and chronically ill children in welfare families. *Journal of Marriage and Family, 62*(2), 399–415.

Lynch, J., Smith, G.D., Harper, S., Hillemeier, M., Ross, N., Kaplan, G.A., & Wolfson, M. (2004). Is income inequality a determinant of population health? Part 1. A systematic review. *The Milbank Quarterly, 82*(1), 5–99. https://doi.org/10.1111/j.0887-378X.2004.00302.x

MacLeod, K.B., & Brownlie, E.B. (2014). Mental health and transitions from adolescence to emerging adulthood: Developmental and diversity considerations. *Canadian Journal of Community Mental Health, 33*(1), 77–86.

Maggi, S., Ostry, A., Callaghan, K., Hershler, R., Chen, L., D'Angiulli, A., & Hertzman, C. (2010). Rural-urban migration patterns and mental health diagnoses of adolescents and young adults in British Columbia, Canada: A case-control study. *Child and Adolescent Psychiatry and Mental Health, 4*(1), 13. https://doi.org/10.1186/1753-2000-4-13. Medline:20465838

Maimann, K. (2014, August 8). Somali youth struggles discussed. *Edmonton Sun.* https://edmontonsun.com/2014/08/08/somali-youth-struggles-discussed /wcm/efc45576-8bb2-4c7b-b77e-e20827e2cc81

Maina, G., Phaneuf, T., Kennedy, M., Mclean, M., Gakumo, A., Nguemo, J., ... Mcharo, S.K. (2020). School-based interventions for preventing substance use in indigenous children ages 7–13: A scoping review protocol. *BMJ Open, 10*(2), e034032. https://doi.org/10.1136/bmjopen-2019-034032. Medline:32051315

Makwarimba, E., Stewart, M., Simich, L., Makumbe, K., Shizha, E., & Anderson, S. (2013). Sudanese and Somali refugees in Canada: Social support needs and preferences. *International Migration, 51*(5), 106–19. https://doi.org /10.1111/imig.12116

Makwarimba, M.J., Kushner, K.E., Letourneau, N.L., Dennis, C., & Shihza, E. (2017). Social support needs and preferences of Sudanese and Zimbabwean refugee new parents in Canada. *International Journal of Migration, Health, and Social Care, 13*(2), 234–52. https://doi.org/10.1108/IJMHSC-07-2014 -0028

Mangham, C., Reid, G., & Stewart, M. (1996). Resilience in families: Challenges for health promotion. *Canadian Journal of Public, 87*(6), 373–4. https://www.jstor.org/stable/41993833

Marmot, M. (2007). Achieving health equity: From root causes to fair outcomes. *The Lancet, 370*(9593), 1153–63. https://doi.org/10.1016/S0140-6736(07)61385-3. Medline:17905168

Marques, L., Leblanc, N.J., Weingarden, H.M., Timpano, K.R., Jenike, M., & Wilhelm, S. (2010). Barriers to treatment and service utilization in an internet sample of individuals with obsessive-compulsive symptoms. *Depression and Anxiety, 27*(5), 470–5. https://doi.org/10.1002/da.20694. Medline:20455248

Marsh, T.N., Marsh, D.C., Ozawagosh, J., & Ozawagosh, F. (2018). The Sweat Lodge Ceremony: A healing intervention for intergenerational trauma and substance use. *International Indigenous Policy Journal, 9*(2). https://doi.org/10.18584/iipj.2018.9.2.2

Marshall, E.A., Butler, K., Roche, T., Cumming, J., & Taknint, J.T. (2016). Refugee youth: A review of mental health counselling issues and practices. *Canadian Psychiatry, 57*(4), 308–19. https://doi.org/10.1037/cap0000068

Martin, D., Miller, A.P., Quesnel- Vallée, A., Caron, N.R., Vissandjée, B., & Marchildon, G.P. (2018). Canada's universal health-care system: Achieving its potential. *Lancet, 391*, 1718–35. https://doi.org/10.1016/50140-6736(18)30181-8. Medline:29483027

Masten A.S. (2012). *Realizing the potential of immigrant youth.* Cambridge University Press.

Mataix-Cols, D., Boman, M., Monzani, B., Ruck, C., Serlachius, E., Langstrom, N., & Lichtenstein, P. (2013). Population-based, multigenerational family clustering study of obsessive-compulsive disorder. *JAMA Psychiatry, 70*(7), 709–17. https://doi.org/10.1001/jamapsychiatry.2013.3. Medline:23699935

Mataix-Cols, D., Frans, E., Pérez-Vigil, A., Kuja-Halkola, R., Gromark, C., Isomura, K., ... Larsson, H. (2017). A total-population multigenerational family clustering study of autoimmune diseases in obsessive-compulsive disorder and Tourette's/chronic tic disorders. *Molecular Psychiatry, 23*(7), 1652–8. https://doi.org/10.1038/mp.2017.215. Medline:29133949

Matsunaga, H., Maebayashi, K., Hayashida, K., Okino, K., Matsui, T., Iketani, T., Kiriike, N., & Stein, D.J. (2008). Symptom structure in Japanese patients with obsessive-compulsive disorder. *American Journal of Psychiatry, 165*(2), 251–3. https://doi.org/10.1176/appi.ajp.2007.07020340. Medline:18006873

Maunder, R.G., Wiesenfeld, L., Lawson, A., & Hunter, J.J. (2019). The relationship between childhood adversity and other aspects of clinical complexity in psychiatric outpatients. *Journal of Interpersonal Violence, 42*, 886260519865968. https://doi.org/10.1177/0886260519865968. Medline:31339443

Mayo, R. (2018). *Impact of family separation in refugee populations.* University of Virginia, School of Medicine. https://med.virginia.edu/family-medicine /wp-content/uploads/sites/285/2018/10/Refugee-Family-Separation-Mayo _Final-092018.pdf

McClure, P. (2000) *Participation support for a more equitable society: Final report of the reference group on welfare reform.* Department of Family and Community Services.

McDermott, S., Dealberto, M.J., DesMeules, M., Kazanjian, A., Manuel, D., Ruddick, E., & Vissandjee, B. (2007, November 15). *Psychoses-related acute hospital discharges among immigrants arriving to Canada between 1985 and 2000: A linkage follow-up study using administrative data* [Poster presentation]. Proceedings of the Canadian Academy of Psychiatric Epidemiology conference.

McGhan, S.L., Cicutto, L.C., & Befus, A.D. (2005). Advances in development and evaluation of asthma education programs. *Current Opinion in Pulmonary Medicine, 11*(1), 61–8. https://doi.org/10.1097/01.mcp.0000146783.18716.31. Medline:15591890

McKenzie, K., Agic, B., Tuck, A., & Antwi M. (2016). *The case for diversity: Building the case to improve mental health services for immigrant, refugee, ethno-cultural and racialized populations.* Report to the Mental Health Commission of Canada. www.mentalhealthcommission.ca/sites/default/files/2016-10 /case_for_diversity_oct_2016_eng.pdf

Mechakra-Tahiri, S., Zunzunegui, M.V. & Seguin, L. (2008). Self-rated health and postnatal depressive symptoms among immigrant mothers in Quebec. *Women's Health, 45*(4), 1–17. https://doi.org/10.1300/J013v45n04_01. Medline:18032165

Medeiros, G.C., Torres, A.R., Boisseau, C.L., Leppink, E.W., Eisen, J.L., Fontenelle, L.F., … Grant, J.E. (2017). A cross-cultural clinical comparison between subjects with obsessive-compulsive disorder from the United States and Brazil. *Psychiatry Research, 254,* 104–11. https://doi.org/10.1016 /j.psychres.2017.04.024. Medline:28457988

Melchior, M., Chastang, J.-F., Falissard, B., Galéra, C., Tremblay, R.E., Côté, S.M., & Boivin, M. (2012). Food insecurity and children's mental health: A prospective birth cohort study. *PLoS ONE, 7*(12), e52615. https://doi.org /10.1371/journal.pone.0052615. Medline:23300723

Menezes, N.M., Georgiades, K., & Boyle, M.H. (2011). The influence of immigrant status and concentration on psychiatric disorder in Canada: A multi-level analysis. *Psychological Medicine, 41*(10), 2221–31. https://doi .org/1017/S0033291711000213. Medline:21349240

Mensah, J., & Williams, C.J. (2013). Ghanaian and Somali immigrants in Toronto's rental market: A comparative cultural perspective of housing issues and coping strategies. *Canadian Ethnic Studies, 45*(1), 115–41. https://doi.org/10.1353/ces.2013.0013

Mental Health Commission of Canada (MHCC). (2013). *Making the case for investing in mental health in Canada.* www.mentalhealthcommission.ca/sites/default/files/2016-06/Investing_in_Mental_Health_FINAL_Version_ENG.pdf

Mental Health Commission of Canada (MHCC). (2018). *Expanding access to psychotherapy: Mapping lessons learned from Australia and the United Kingdom to the Canadian context.* https://www.mentalhealthcommission.ca/sites/default/files/2018-08/Expanding_Access_to_Psychotherapy_2018.pdf

Micali, N., Heyman, I., Perez, M., Hilton, K., Nakatani, E., Turner, C., & Mataix-Cols, D. (2010). Long-term outcomes of obsessive-compulsive disorder: Follow-up of 142 children and adolescents. *British Journal of Psychiatry, 197*(2), 128–34. https://doi.org/10.1192/bjp.bp.109.075317. Medline:20679265

Mi'kmaw Ethics Watch. (1999). *Research principles and protocols.* Cape Breton University.

Mitschke, D.B., Praetorius, R.T., Kelly, D.R., Small, E., & Kim, Y.K. (2017). Listening to refugees: How traditional mental health interventions may miss the mark. *International Social Work, 60*(3): 588–600. https://doi.org/10.1177/0020872816648256

Molm, L.D. (1997). *Coercive power in social exchange.* Cambridge University Press.

Mood Disorders Society of Canada (2007). *Quick facts: Mental illness and addiction in Canada.* Mood Disorders Society of Canada. www.mooddisorderscanada.ca/documents/Media%20Room/Quick%20Facts%203rd%20Edition%20Eng%20Nov%2012%2009.pdf

Moore, T.G., McDonald, M., Carlon, L., & O'Rourke, K. (2015). Early childhood development and the social determinants of health inequities. *Health Promotion International, 30*(Suppl. 2), 102–15. https://doi.org/10.1093/heapro/dav031. Medline:26420806

Murphy, J.M., Guzman, J., McCarthy, A.E., Squicciarini, A.M., George, M., Canenguez, K.M., ... Jellinek, M.S. (2015). Mental health predicts better academic outcomes: A longitudinal study of elementary school students in Chile. *Child Psychiatry & Human Development, 46*(2), 245–56. https://doi.org/10.1007/s10578-014-0464-4. Medline:24771270

Murray, C.J., & Lopez, A.D. (1997). Global mortality, disability, and the contribution of risk factors: Global burden of disease study. *Lancet, 349*(9063), 1436–42. https://doi.org/10.1016/S0140-6736(96)07495-8. Medline:9164317

Nagata, J.M., Weiser, S.D., Gooding, H.C., Garber, A.K., Bibbins-Domingo, K., & Palar, K. (2019, June 24). Association between food insecurity and migraine among US young adults [research letter]. *JAMA Neurology.* https://doi.org/10.1001/jamaneurol.2019.1663. Medline:31233123

Nasreen, S., Brar, R., Brar, S., Maltby, A., & Wilk, P. (2018). Are Indigenous determinants of health associated with self-reported health professional-diagnosed anxiety disorders among Canadian First Nations adults? Findings from the 2012 Aboriginal Peoples survey. *Community Mental Health Journal, 54*(4), 460–8. https://doi.org/10.1007/s10597-017-0165-0. Medline:28887731

National Collaborating Centre for Aboriginal Health (NCCAH). (2012). *The state of knowledge of Aboriginal health: A review of Aboriginal public health in Canada.* www.ccnsa-nccah.ca/docs/context/RPT-StateKnowledgeReview-EN.pdf

National Collaborating Centre for Aboriginal Health (NCCAH). (2013). *Setting the context: An overview of Aboriginal health in Canada.* University of Northern British Columbia. www.nccah-ccnsa.ca

National Collaborating Centre for Aboriginal Health (NCCAH). (2017). *Social determinants of health: Tackling poverty in Indigenous communities in Canada.* www.ccnsa-nccah.ca/docs/determinants/FS-TacklingPovertyCanada-SDOH-Wien-EN.pdf

Negreiros, J., Belschner, L., Selles, R.R., Lin, S., & Stewart, S.E. (2018). Academic skills in pediatric obsessive-compulsive disorder: A preliminary study. *Annals of Clinical Psychiatry, 30*(3), 185–95. Medline:30028892

Nelson, S.E., & Wilson, K. (2018). Understanding barriers to health care access through cultural safety and ethical space: Indigenous people's experiences in Prince George, Canada. *Social Science and Medicine, 218*, 21–7. https://doi.org/10.1016/j.socscimed.2018.09.017. Medline:30316132

Nestadt, G., Bienvenu, O.J., Cai, G., Samuels, J., & Eaton, W.W. (1998). Incidence of obsessive-compulsive disorder in adults. *Journal of Nervous & Mental Disease, 186*(7), 401–6. https://doi.org/10.1097/00005053-199807000-00003. Medline:9680040

Nestadt, G., Samuels, J., Riddle, M., Bienvenu, O. J., Liang, K. Y., LaBuda, M., … Hoehn-Saric, R. (2000). A family study of obsessive-compulsive disorder. *Archives of General Psychiatry, 57*(4), 358–63. https://doi.org/10.1001/archpsyc.57.4.358

Nettleton, C., Napolitano, D.A., & Stephens, C. (2007). *An overview of current knowledge of the social determinants of Indigenous health.* Commission on the Social Determinants of Health, World Health Organization. https://researchonline.lshtm.ac.uk/id/eprint/6662/1/An%20Overview%20of%20Current%20Knowledge%20of%20the%20Social%20Determinants%20of%20Indigenous%20Health%20Working%20Paper.pdf

Nicolini, H., Salin-Pascual, R., Cabrera, B., & Lanzagorta, N. (2017). Influence of culture in obsessive-compulsive disorder and its treatment. *Current Psychiatry Reviews, 13*(4), 285–92. https://doi.org/10.2174/2211556007666180115105935. Medline:29657563

O'Donnell, S., Syoufi, M., Jones, W., Bennett, K., & Pelletier, L. (2017). Use of medication and psychological counselling among Canadians with mood and/ or anxiety disorders. *Health Promotion & Chronic Disease Prevention in Canada, 37*(5), 160–71. https://doi.org/10.24095/hpcdp.37.5.04. Medline:28493660

Ontario Association of Children's Aid Societies (2015). One vision one voice: Changing the child welfare system for African Canadians. http://www .oacas.org/wp-content/uploads/2015/09/Workbook-African-Canadians -Project-August-2015.pdf

Ontario Institute for Studies in Education. (2020). *Indigenous ways of knowing.* University of Toronto. https://www.oise.utoronto.ca/abed101/indigenous -ways-of-knowing

Opoku-Dapaah, E. (2006). African immigrants in Canada: Trends, socio-demographic and spatial aspects. In K. Konadu-Agyemang, B.K. Takyi, & J.A. Arthur (Eds.), *The new African diaspora in North America: Trends, community building, and adaptation* (pp. 69–93). Lexington Books.

Orlovska, S., Vestergaard, C.H., Bech, B.H., Nordentoft, M., Vestergaard, M., & Benros, M.E. (2017). Association of streptococcal throat infection with mental disorders: Testing key aspects of the PANDAS hypothesis in a nationwide study. *JAMA Psychiatry, 74*(7), 740–6. https://doi.org/10.1001 /jamapsychiatry.2017.0995. Medline:28538981

Osland, S., Arnold, P.D., & Pringsheim, T. (2018). The prevalence of diagnosed obsessive compulsive disorder and associated comorbidities: A population-based Canadian study. *Psychiatry Research, 268,* 137–42. https://doi.org /10.1016/j.psychres.2018.07.018. Medline:30025284

Ostrowski, S.A., Christopher, N.C., & Delahanty, D.L. (2007). Brief report: the impact of maternal posttraumatic stress disorder symptoms and child gender on risk for persistent posttraumatic stress disorder symptoms in child trauma victims. *Journal of Pediatric Psychology, 32*(3), 338–42. https://doi.org /10.1093/jpepsy/jsl006. Medline:16717137

Oxman-Martinez, J., Rummens, A.J., Moreau, J., Choi, Y.R., Beiser, M., Ogilvie, L., & Armstrong, R. (2012). Perceived ethnic discrimination and social exclusion: Newcomer immigrant children in Canada. *American Journal Orthopsychiatry, 82*(3), 376–88. https://doi.org/10.1111/j.1939-0025 .2012.01161.x. Medline:22880976

Pahwa, P., Abonyi, S., Karunanayake, C., Rennie, D.C., Janzen, B., Kirychuk, S., ... Dosman, J.A. (2015). A community-based participatory research methodology to address, redress, and reassess disparities in respiratory health among First Nations. *BMC Research Notes, 8*(199). https://doi.org /10.1186s13104-015-1137-5. Medline:25981585

Pahwa, P., Karunanayake, C.P., McCrosky, J., & Thorpe, L. (2012). Longitudinal trends in mental health among ethnic groups in Canada. *Chronic Diseases and Injuries in Canada, 32*(3), 164–76. Medline:22762903

Pahwa, P., Karunanayake, C.P., Rennie, D.C., Lawson, J.A., Ramsden, V.R., McMullin, K., ... Dosman, J.A. (2017). Prevalence and associated risk factors of chronic bronchitis in First Nations people. *BMC Pulmonary Medicine, 17*(1). https://doi.org/10.1186/s12890-017-0432-4. Medline:28662706

Palardy, V., El-Baalbaki, G., Fredette, C., Rizkallah, E., & Guay, S. (2018). Social support and symptom severity among patients with obsessive-compulsive disorder or panic disorder with agoraphobia: A systematic review. *European Journal of Psychology, 14*(1), 254–86. https://doi.org/10.5964/ejop.v14i1.1252. Medline:29899808

Paradies, Y., Priest, N., Ben, J., Truong, M., Gupta, A., Pieterse, A., Kelaher, M., & Gee, G. (2013). Racism as a determinant of health: A protocol for conducting a systematic review and meta-analysis. *Systematic Reviews, 2,* 85. https://doi.org/10.1186/2046-4053-2-85. Medline:24059279

Patten, S. (2019). The 2014 Ontario Child Health Study. *Canadian Journal of Psychiatry, 64*(4), 225–6. https://doi.org/10.1177/0706743719834483. Medline:30978143

Patterson, B., Kyu, H.H., & Georgiades, K. (2013). Age at immigration to Canada and the occurrence of mood, anxiety, and substance use disorders. *Canadian Journal of Psychiatry, 58*(4), 210–17. https://doi.org/10.1177/070674371305800406. Medline:23547644

Pearce, A., Dundas, R., Whitehead, M., & Taylor-Robinson, D. (2019). Pathways to inequalities in child health. *Archives of Disease in Childhood, 9*(104), 998–1003. https://doi.org/10.1136/archdischild-2018-314808.

Pediatric OCD Treatment Study Team. (2004). Cognitive-behavior therapy, sertraline, and their combination for children and adolescents with obsessive-compulsive disorder: The Pediatric OCD Treatment Study (POTS) randomized controlled trial. *JAMA, 292*(16), 1969–76. https://doi.org/10.1001/jama.292.16.1969. Medline:15507582

Pérez-Vigil, A., Fernández de la Cruz, L., Brander, G., Isomura, K., Jangmo, A., Feldman, I., ... Mataix-Cols, D. (2018). Association of obsessive-compulsive disorder with objective indicators of educational attainment: A nationwide register-based sibling control study. *JAMA Psychiatry, 75*(1), 47–55. https://doi.org/10.1001/jamapsychiatry.2017.3523. Medline:29141084

Peris, T.S., & Miklowitz, D.J. (2015). Parental expressed emotion and youth psychopathology: New directions for an old construct. *Child Psychiatry & Human Development, 46*(6), 863–73. https://doi.org/10.1007/s10578-014-0526-7. Medline:25552241

Peris, T.S., Rozenman, M.S., Sugar, C.A., McCracken, J.T., & Piacentini, J. (2017). Targeted family intervention for complex cases of pediatric obsessive-compulsive disorder: A randomized controlled trial. *Journal of the American Academy of Child & Adolescent Psychiatry, 56*(12), 1034–42.e1031. https://doi.org/10.1016/j.jaac.2017.10.008. Medline:29173737

Peris, T.S., Sugar, C.A., Bergman, R.L., Chang, S., Langley, A., & Piacentini, J. (2012). Family factors predict treatment outcome for pediatric obsessive-compulsive disorder. *Journal of Consulting & Clinical Psychology, 80*(2), 255–63. https://doi.org/10.1037/a0027084 10.1037/a0027084. Medline:22309471

Peters, I., Handley, T., Oakley, K., Lutkin, S., & Perkins, D. (2019). Social determinants of psychological wellness for children and adolescents in rural NSW. *BMC Public Health, 19*(1), 1616. https://doi.org/10.1186/s12889-019 -7961-0. Medline:31791290

Petrucka, P., Bickford, D., Bassendowski, S., Goodwill, W., Wajunta, C., Yuzicappi, B. ... Rauliuk, M. (2016). Positive leadership, legacy, lifestyles, attitudes, and activities for Aboriginal youth: A wise practices approach for positive Aboriginal youth futures. *International Journal of Indigenous Health, 11*(1), 177–97.

Phillips-Beck, W., Eni, R., Lavoie, J., Avery Kinew, K., Kyoon Achan, G. & Katz, R. (2020). Confronting racism within the Canadian health care system: Systemic exclusion of First Nations from quality and consistent care. *International Journal of Environment Research in Public Health, 17*(22), 8343. https//doi.org/10.3390/ijerph17228343

Piacentini, J., Bergman, R.L., Keller, M., & McCracken, J. (2003). Functional impairment in children and adolescents with obsessive-compulsive disorder. *Journal of Child & Adolescent Psychopharmacology, 13*(Suppl. 2), S61–9. https:// doi.org/10.1089/104454603322126359. Medline:12880501

Piacentini, J., Peris, T.S., Bergman, R.L., Chang, S., & Jaffer, M. (2007). Functional impairment in childhood OCD: Development and psychometrics properties of the Child Obsessive-Compulsive Impact Scale-Revised (COIS-R). *Journal of Clinical Child & Adolescent Psychology, 36*(4), 645–53. https://doi.org/10.1080/15374410701662790. Medline:18088221

Pieloch, K.A., McCullough, M.B., & Marks, A.K. (2016). Resilience of children with refugee statuses: A research review. *Canadian Psychology, 57*(4), 330–9. https://doi.org/10.1037/cap0000073

Pitt, R.S., Sherman, J., & Macdonald, M.E. (2016). Low-income working immigrant families in Quebec: Exploring their challenges to well-being. *Canadian Journl of Public Health, 106*(8), e539–45. Medline:26986917

Pocock, N., & Chan, C. (2018). Refugees, racism and xenophobia: What works to reduce discrimination? *Our World.* United Nations University. https:// ourworld.unu.edu/en/refugees-racism-and-xenophobia-what-works-to -reduce-discrimination

Postl, B.D., Cook, C.L., & Moffatt, M. (2010). Aboriginal child health and the social determinants: Why are these children so disadvantaged? *Healthcare Quarterly, 14*(Sp), 42–51. https://doi.org/10.12927/hcq.2010.21982. Medline:20959746

Poureslami, I., Nimmon, L., Rootman, I., & Fitzgerald, M.J. (2017). Health literacy and chronic disease management: Drawing from expert knowledge to set an agenda. *Health Promotion International, 32*(4), 743–54. https://doi .org/10.1093/heapro/daw003. Medline:26873913

Poyraz, C.A., Turan, Ş., Sağlam, N.G.U., Batun, G.Ç., Yassa, A., & Duran, A. (2015). Factors associated with the duration of untreated illness among patients with obsessive compulsive disorder. *Comprehensive Psychiatry, 58*, 88–93. https://doi.org/10.1016/j.comppsych.2014.12.019. Medline:25596625

Protudjer, J.L.P, Kozyrskyj, A.L., & Becker, A.B. (2011). *Asthma is a low priority amidst the layers of complexity faced by adolescents.* [Paper presentation]. AllerGen NCE.

Protudjer, J.L.P, Kozyrskyj, A.L., Becker, A.B., & Marchessault, G. (2009). Normalization strategies of children with asthma. *Qualitative Health Research, 19*(1), 94–104. https://doi.org/10.1177/1049732308327348. Medline:18997151

Przeworski, A., Zoellner, L.A., Franklin, M.E., Garcia, A., Freeman, J., March, J.S., & Foa, E.B. (2012). Maternal and child expressed emotion as predictors of treatment response in pediatric obsessive-compulsive disorder. *Child Psychiatry & Human Development, 43*(3), 337–53. https://doi.org/10.1007 /s10578-011-0268-8. Medline:22090186

Public Health Agency of Canada (PHAC). (2008). *The Chief Public Health Officer's report on the state of public health in Canada.* Government of Canada. www.phac-aspc.gc.ca/cphorsphc-respcacsp/2008/fr-rc/index-eng.php

Public Health Agency of Canada (PHAC). (2018). *Key health inequalities in Canada: A national portrait.* Government of Canada.

Public Safety Canada. (2007). *Youth gangs in Canada: What do we know?* Government of Canada. https://www.publicsafety.gc.ca/cnt/rsrcs/pblctns /gngs-cnd/gngs-cnd-eng.pdf

Raphael, D. (2006, July 1). *Politics, political platforms and child poverty in Canada.* Policy Options. https://policyoptions.irpp.org/fr/magazines/border -security/politics-political-platforms-and-child poverty-in-canada

Raphael, D. (2007). *Poverty and policy in Canada.*Canadian Scholars' Press.

Raphael, D. (2008). Getting serious about the social determinants of health: New directions for public health workers. *IUHPE Promotion and Education, 15*(3), 15–20. https://doi.org/10.1177/1025382308095650. Medline:18784048

Raphael, D. (2010). The health of Canada's children. Part IV: Toward the future. *Paediatric Child Health, 15*(4), 199–204. https://doi.org/10.1093 /pch/15.4.199. Medline:21455463

Raphael, D. (2014). Social determinants of children's health in Canada: Analysis and implications. *International Journal of Child, Youth and Family Studies, 5*(2), 220–39. https://doi.org/10.18357/ijcyfs.raphaeld.522014

Reading, C. & Wien, F. (2009). *Health inequities and social determinants of Aboriginal peoples' health.* National Collaborating Centre for Aboriginal Health.

Redvers, N., Marianayagam, J., & Be'sha Blondin. (2019). Improving access to Indigenous medicine for patients in hospital-based settings: A challenge for health systems in northern Canada. International Journal of Circumpolar Health, *78*(1). https://doi.org/10.1080/22423982.2019.1577093. Medline:30744519

Refugee health is a crisis of our own making. (2019). *The Lancet, 393*(10191), 2563. https://doi.org/10.1016/S0140-6736(19)31423-0

Reid, A.M., Guzick, A.G., Fernandez, A.G., Deacon, B., McNamara, J.P.H., Geffken, G.R., ... Striley, C.W. (2018). Exposure therapy for youth with anxiety: Utilization rates and predictors of implementation in a sample of practicing clinicians from across the United States. *Journal of Anxiety Disorders, 58,* 8–17. https://doi.org/10.1016/j.janxdis.2018.06.002. Medline:29929139

Reiss, F. (2013). Socioeconomic inequalities and mental health problems in children and adolescents: A systematic review. *Social Science and Medicine, 90,* 24–31. https://doi.org/10.1016/j.socscimed.2013.04.026. Medline:23746605

Reutter, L., Stewart, M.J., Raine, K., Williamson, D., Letourneau, N., & McFall, S. (2005). Partnerships and participation in conducting poverty-related health research. *Primary Health Care Research and Development, 6*(4), 356–66. https://doi.org/10.1191/1463423605pc260oa

Richmond, C.A.M. (2007). Narratives of social support and health in Aboriginal communities. *Canadian Journal of Public Health, 98*(4), 347–51. https://doi.org/10.1007/BF03405416. Medline:17896750

Richmond, C.A.M., & Cook, C. (2016). Creating conditions for Canadian aboriginal equity: The promise of healthy public policy. *Public Health Reviews, 37*(2), 1–16. https://doi.org/10.1186/s40985-016-0016-5. Medline:29450044

Rintala, H., Chudal, R., Leppämäki, S., Leivonen, S., Hinkka-Yli-Salomäki, S., & Sourander, A. (2017). Register-based study of the incidence, comorbidities and demographics of obsessive-compulsive disorder in specialist healthcare. *BMC Psychiatry, 17*(1), 64. https://doi.org/10.1186/s12888-017-1224-3. Medline:28183286

Robinson, C. (2019). The impact of poverty on Canadian children: A call for action. *CMAJ Blogs.* https://cmajblogs.com/the-impact-of-poverty-on-canadian-children-a-call-for-action/

Rogers, B.J., Swift, K., van der Woerd, K., Auger, M., Halseth, R., Atkinson, D., ... Bedard, A. (2019). *At the interface: Indigenous health practitioners and evidence-based practice.* National Collaborating Centre for Aboriginal Health. www.nccah-ccnsa.ca/docs/context/RPT-At-the-Interface-Halseth-EN.pdf

Rosychuk, R.J., Voaklander, D.C., Klassen, T.P., Senthilselvan, A., Marrie, T.J., & Rowe, B.H. (2010a). Asthma presentations by children to emergency departments in a Canadian province: A population-based study. *Pediatric*

Pulmonology, 45(10), 985–92. https://doi.org/10.1002/ppul.21281. Medline:20632409

Rosychuk, R.J., Voaklander, D.C., Klassen, T.R., Senthilselvan, A., Marrie, T.J., & Rowe, B.H. (2010b). A population-based study of emergency department presentations for asthma in regions of Alberta. *Canadian Journal of Emergency Medicine, 12*(4), 339–46. https://doi.org/10.1017/S1481803500012434. Medline:20650027

Ruscio, A.M., Stein, D.J., Chiu, W.T., & Kessler, R.C. (2010). The epidemiology of obsessive-compulsive disorder in the National Comorbidity Survey Replication. *Molecular Psychiatry, 15*(1), 53–63. https://doi.org/10.1038/mp.2008.94. Medline:18725912

Russell, A.E., Ford, T., Williams, R., & Russell, G. (2016). The association between socioeconomic disadvantage and attention deficit/hyperactivity disorder (ADHD): A systematic review. *Child Psychiatry & Human Development, 47*(3), 440–58. Medline:26266467

Russell, C., Neufeld, M., Sabioni, P., Varatharajan, T., Ali, F., Miles, S., ... Rehm, J. (2019). Assessing service and treatment needs and barriers of youth who use illicit and non-medical prescription drugs in Northern Ontario, Canada. *PLoS ONE, 14*(12), e0225548. https://doi.org/10.1371/journal.pone.0225548. Medline:31805082

Russell, D.W. (1996). UCLA Loneliness Scale (version 3): Reliability, validity, and factor structure. *Journal of Personality Assessment, 66*(1), 20–40. https://doi.org/10.1207/s15327752jpa6601_2. Medline:8576833

Saddichha, S., Torchalla, I., & Krausz, M.R. (2014). Gender differences in early trauma and high-risk behaviors among street-entrenched youth in British Columbia. *Interntional Journal of Adolescent Medicine & Health, 26*(4), 489–93. https://doi.org/10.1515/ijamh-2013-0323. Medline:24447985

*Sadock, B.J., & Sadock, V.A. (2002). *Synopsis of psychiatry: Behavioral sciences/ clinical psychiatry* (9th ed.). Lippincott Williams & Wilkins.

Salami, B., Hegadoren, K., Bautista, L., Ben-Shlomo, Y., Diaz, E., Rammohan, A., ... Yaskina, M. (2017). *Mental health of immigrants and non-immigrants in Canada: Evidence from the Canadian Health Measures Survey and Service Provider Interviews in Alberta.* PolicyWise for Children and Families. https://policywise.com/wp-content/uploads/resources/2017/04/2017-04APR-27-Scientific-Report-15SM-SalamiHegadoren.pdf

Salami, B., Okeke-Ihejirika, P., Yohani, S., Vallianatos, H., Nsaliwa, C., Ayalew, T., & Alaazi, D. (2017). *Parenting and mental health promotion practices of African immigrants in Alberta.* Submitted to stakeholders, including Alberta Minister of Health; Parliamentary Secretary to the Minister of Heritage; Immigration, Refugee and Citizenship Canada. https://era.library.ualberta.ca/files/b7h149q08m#.WnZ9vqinE2w

Salami, B., Yaskina, M., Hegadoren, K., Diaz, E., Meherali, S., Rammohan, A., & Ben-Shlomo, Y. (2017). Migration and social determinants of mental health: Results from the Canadian Health Measures Survey. *Canadian Journal of Public Health, 108*(4), 362–7. https://doi.org/10.17269/CJPH.108.6105. Medline:29120306

Saunders, N.R., Gill, P.J., Holder, L., Vigod, S., Kurdyak, P., Gandhi, S., & Guttmann, A. (2018). Use of the emergency department as a first point of contact for mental health care by immigrant youth in Canada: A population-based study. *Canadian Medical Association Journal, 190*(40), E1183–E1191. https://doi.org/10.1503/cmaj.180277. Medline: 30301742

Saunders, N.R., Lebenbaum, M., Lu, H., Stukel, T.A., Urquia, M.L., & Guttmann, A. (2018). Trends in mental health service utilisation in immigrant youth in Ontario, Canada, 1996–2012: A population-based longitudinal cohort study. *BMJ Open, 8*(9), e022647. https://doi.org /10.1136/bmjopen-2018-022647. Medline:30224392

Schaffer, A., Cairney, J., Cheung, A., Veldhuizen, S., Kurdyak, P., & Levitt, A. (2009). Differences in prevalence and treatment of bipolar disorder among immigrants: Results from an epidemiologic survey. *Canadian Journal of Psychiatry, 54*(11), 734–42. https://doi.org/10.1177/070674370905401103. Medline:19961661

Schofield, T. (2007). Health inequity and its social determinants: A sociological commentary. *Health Sociology Review, 16*(2), 105–14. https://doi.org/10.5172 /hesr.2007.16.2.105

Schulze, S. (2003). Views on the combination of quantitative and qualitative research approaches. *Progressio, 25*(2), 8–20. http://hdl.handle.net/10500 /195

Schweitzer, R., Melville, F., Steel., Z., & Lacherez, P. (2006). Trauma, post migration living difficulties, and social support as predictors of psychological adjustment in resettled Sudanese refugees. *Australian and New Zealand Journal of Psychiatry, 40*(2), 179–87. https://doi.org/10.1080/ j.1440-1614.2006.01766.x. Medline:16476137

Selles, R.R., Belschner, L., Negreiros, J., Lin, S., Schuberth, D., McKenney, K., ... Stewart, S.E. (2018). Group family-based cognitive behavioral therapy for pediatric obsessive compulsive disorder: Global outcomes and predictors of improvement. *Psychiatry Research, 260*, 116–22. https://doi.org/10.1016 /j.psychres.2017.11.041. Medline:29179016

Selles, R.R., Franklin, M., Sapyta, J., Compton, S.N., Tommet, D., Jones, R.N., ... Freeman, J. (2018). Children's and parents' ability to tolerate child distress: Impact on cognitive behavioral therapy for pediatric obsessive compulsive disorder. *Child Psychiatry & Human Development, 49*(2), 308–16. https://doi .org/10.1007/s10578-017-0748-6. Medline:28756555

Selles, R.R., Højgaard, D.R.M.A., Ivarsson, T., Thomsen, P.H., McBride, N., Storch, E.A., ... Stewart, S.E. (2018). Symptom insight in pediatric obsessive-compulsive disorder: Outcomes of an international aggregated cross-sectional sample. *Journal of the American Academy of Child & Adolescent Psychiatry, 57*(8), 615–19.e5. https://doi.org/10.1016/j.jaac.2018.04.012. Medline:30071984

Settipani, C.A., Hawke, L.D., Virdo, G., Yorke, E., Mehra, K., & Henderson, J. (2018). Social determinants of health among youth seeking substance use and mental health treatment. *Journal of Canadian Academy of Child and Adolescent Psychiatry, 27*(4), 213–21. Medline:30487936

Sevilla-Cermeño, L., Andrén, P., Hillborg, M., Silverberg-Morse, M., Mataix-Cols, D., & Fernández de la Cruz, L. (2019). Insomnia in pediatric obsessive-compulsive disorder: Prevalence and association with multimodal treatment outcomes in a naturalistic clinical setting. *Sleep Medicine, 56*, 104–10. https://doi.org/10.1016/j.sleep.2018.12.024. Medline:30852130

Sheldon, T.A., & Parker, H. (1992). Race and ethnicity in health research. *Journal of Public Health Medicine, 14*(2), 104–10. https://doi.org/10.1093/oxfordjournals.pubmed.a042706

Shetti, C.N., Reddy, Y.C., Kandavel, T., Kashyap, K., Singisetti, S., Hiremath, A.S., ... Raghunandanan, S. (2005). Clinical predictors of drug nonresponse in obsessive-compulsive disorder. *Journal of Clinical Psychiatry, 66*(12), 1517–23. Medline:16401151

Shields, J., & Lujan, O. (2018). *Immigrant youth in Canada: A literature review of migrant youth settlement and service issues.* CERIS project funded by Immigration, Refugee and Citizenship Canada. http://ceris.ca/IWYS/wp-content/uploads/2018/09/IWYS-Knowledge-Synthesis-Report-Youth-report-Sept-2018.pdf

Shields-Zeeman, L., Lewis, C., & Gottlieb, L. (2019). Social and mental health care integration: The leading edge. *JAMA Psychiatry, 76*(9), 881–2. https://doi.org/10.1001/jamapsychiatry.2019.1148. Medline:31215983

Shimmin, C. (2015). *Five things to know about the relationship between poverty and health in Canada.* Institute for Research in Public Policy. http://policyoptions.irpp.org/2015/10/05/five-things-to-know-about-the-relationship-between-poverty-and-health-in-canada/

Shimmin, C. (2020). Backgrounder: The impact of poverty on health. *Making Evidence Matter.* Evidence Network. http://evidencenetwork.ca/backgrounder-the-impact-of-poverty-on-health/

Sickle, D.V., Morgan, F., & Wright, A.L. (2003). Qualitative study of the use of traditional healing by asthmatic Navajo families. *American Indian & Alaska Native Mental Health Research: The Journal of the National Center, 11*(1), 1–18. https://doi.org/10.5820/aian.1101.2003.1. Medline:12955629

Sidorchuk, A., Kuja-Halkola, R., Runeson, B., Lichtenstein, P., Larsson, H., Rück, C., … Fernández de la Cruz, L. (2019). Genetic and environmental sources of familial coaggregation of obsessive-compulsive disorder and suicidal behavior: A population-based birth cohort and family study. *Molecular Psychiatry*, *124*(06), 300. https://doi.org/10.1038/s41380-019 -0417-1. Medline:30962511

Simich, L., Beiser, M., Stewart, M., & Makwarimba, E. (2005). Providing social support for immigrants and refugees in Canada: Challenges and directions. *Journal of Immigrant Health*, *7*(4), 259–68. https://doi.org/10.1007/s10903 -005-5123-1. Medline:19813292

Simich, L., Este, D., & Hamilton, H. (2010). Meanings of home and mental well-being among Sudanese refugees in Canada. *Ethnicity and Health*, *15*(2), 199–212. https://doi.org/10.1080/13557851003615560. Medline:20306355

Simonds, L.M., & Elliott, S.A. (2001). OCD patients and non-patient groups reporting obsessions and compulsions: Phenomenology, help-seeking, and access to treatment. *British Journal of Medical Psychology*, *74*(4), 431–49. https://doi.org/10.1348/000711201161091. Medline:11780792

Sin, D.D., Svenson, L.W, Cowie, R.L., & Man, S.F. (2003). Can universal access to health care eliminate health inequities between children of poor and non-poor families? A case study of childhood asthma in Alberta. *Chest*, *124*(1), 51–6. https://doi.org/10.1378/chest.124.1.51. Medline:12853501

Sin, D.D., Wells, H., Svenson, L.W. & Man, S.F.P. (2002). Asthma and COPD among Aboriginals in Alberta, Canada. *Chest*, *121*(6), 1841–6. https://doi .org/10.1378/chest.121.6.1841. Medline:12065347

Singh, G.K., & Ghandour, R.M. (2012). Impact of neighborhood social conditions and household socioeconomic status on behavioral problems among US children. *Maternal & Child Health Journal*, *16*(1), 158–69. https:// doi.org/10.1007/s10995-012-1005-z. Medline:22481571

Skoog, G., & Skoog, I. (1999). A 40-year follow-up of patients with obsessive-compulsive disorder. *Archives of General Psychiatry*, *56*(2), 121–7. https:// doi.org/10.1001/archpsyc.56.2.121. Medline:10025435

Sookman, D., & Fineberg, N.A. (2015). Specialized psychological and pharmacological treatments for obsessive-compulsive disorder throughout the lifespan: A special series by the Accreditation Task Force of the Canadian Institute for Obsessive Compulsive Disorders. *Psychiatry Research*, *227*(1), 74–7. https://doi.org/10.1016/j.psychres.2014.12.002. Medline:25661530

Spencer, A.E., Baul, T.D., Sikov, J., Adams, W.G., Tripodis, Y., Buonocore, O., … Garg, A. (2020). The relationship between social risks and the mental health of school-age children in primary care. *Academic Pediatrics*, *20*(2), 208–15. https://doi.org/10.1016/j.acap.2019.11.006. Medline:31751774

Spencer, N., Raman, S., O'Hare, B., & Tamburlini, G. (2019). Addressing inequities in child health and development: Towards social justice.

BMJ Paediatrics Open, 3(1), e000503. https://doi.org/10.1136/bmjpo-2019
-000503. Medline:31423469

Stafford, M., Newbold, B.K., & Ross, N.A. (2011). Psychological distress
among immigrants and visible minorities in Canada: A contextual analysis.
International Journal of Social Psychiatry, 57(4), 428–41. https://doi.org
/10.1177/0020764010365407. Medline:20378661

Standing Senate Committee on Human Rights. (2007). *Children: The silenced
citizens. Effective implementation of Canada's international obligations with respect to
the rights of children.* www.parl.gc.ca/content/sen/committee/391/huma
/rep/rep10apr07-e.pdf

Statistics Canada. (2013a). *Persons with asthma, by age and sex.* www.statcan
.gc.ca/tables-tableaux/sum-som/l01/cst01/health49a-eng.htm

Statistics Canada. (2013b). *Aboriginal peoples in Canada: First Nations people, Métis
and Inuit.* http://www12.statcan.gc.ca/nhs-enm/2011/as-sa/99-011-x/99
-011-x2011001- eng.pdf

Statistics Canada. (2013c). *Income in Canada, 2011* (CANSIM Table 202-0804).
www5.statcan.gc.ca/cansim/pick-choisir?lang=eng&p2=33&id=2020804

Statistics Canada. (2013d). *Low-income lines, 2010–2011.* www.statcan.gc.ca
/pub/75f0002m/75f0002m2012002-eng.htm

Statistics Canada. (2015). *Low income lines, 2012–2013:* Low income cut-offs.
www150.statcan.gc.ca/n1/pub/75f0002m/2014003/lico-sfr-eng.htm

Statistics Canada. (2016a) *Census of population.* https://www150.statcan.gc.ca
/n1/en/catalogue/98-400-X2016206

Statistics Canada. (2016b) *Census of population.* https://www12.statcan.gc.ca
/census-recensement/2016/dp-pd/dt-td/Rp-eng.cfm?LANG=E&APATH=3&
DETAIL=0&DIM=0&FL=A&FREE=0&GC=0&GID=0&GK=0&GRP=1&PID
=111095&PRID=10&PTYPE=109445&S=0&SHOWALL=0&SUB=0&Temporal
=2017&THEME=122&VID=0&VNAMEE=&VNAMEF=11

Statistics Canada. (2017a). *Immigration and ethnocultural diversity: Key results from
the 2016 census.* www.statcan.gc.ca/daily-quotidien/171025/dq171025b
-eng.htm

Statistics Canada. (2017b). *Census in brief: Children living in low-income households.*
www12.statcan.gc.ca/census-recensement/2016/as-sa/98-200-x/2016012/98
-200-x2016012-eng.cfm

Statistics Canada. (2018a). *The income of Canadians: Median after-tax income of
families and unattached individuals, 2016.* www150.statcan.gc.ca/n1/pub
/11-627-m/11-627-m2018006-eng.htm

Statistics Canada. (2018b). *First Nations people, Metis and Inuit in Canada: Diverse
and growing populations.* https://www150.statcan.gc.ca/n1/pub/89-659-x/89
-659-x2018001-eng.htm

Statistics Canada. (2019). Aboriginal identity (9), income statistics (17),
Registered or Treaty Indian Status (3), age (9) and sex (3) for the population

aged 15 years and over in private households of Canada, provinces and territories, census metropolitan areas and census agglomerations, 2016 Census – 25% sample data. https://www12.statcan.gc.ca/census-recensement/2016/dp-pd/dt-td/Rp-eng.cfm?LANG=E&APATH=3&DETAIL=0&DIM=0&FL=A&FREE=0&GC=0&GID=0&GK=0&GRP=1&PID=110523&PRID=10&PTYPE=109445&S=0&SHOWALL=0&SUB=0&Temporal=2017&THEME=122&VID=0&VNAMEE=&VNAMEF=FROM

Stengler-Wenzke, K., Kroll, M., Matschinger, H., & Angermeyer, M.C. (2006). Quality of life of relatives of patients with obsessive-compulsive disorder. *Comprehensive Psychiatry, 47*(6), 523–7. https://doi.org/10.1016/j.comppsych.2006.02.002. Medline:17067878

Stewart, L., & Nielsen, A-M. (2011). Two Aboriginal registered nurses show us why Black nurses caring for Black patients is good medicine. *Contemporary Nurse, 37*(1), 96–101. https://doi.org/10.5172/conu.2011.37.1.096. Medline:21591832

Stewart, M. (2000). Social support, coping, and self-care as public participation mechanisms. In M.J. Stewart (Ed.), *Community nursing: Promoting Canadians' health* (2nd ed., pp. 83–104). W.B. Saunders Company.

Stewart, M., Anderson, J., Beiser, M., Makwarimba, E., Neufeld, A., Simich, L. & Spitzer, S. (2008). Multicultural meanings of social support among immigrants and refugees. *International Migration, 46*(3), 123–59. https://doi.org/10.1111/j.1468-2435.2008.00464.x

Stewart, M., Barnfather, A., Magill-Evans, J., Ray, L., Letourneau, N., & Erickson, D. (2011). Brief report – An online support intervention: Perceptions of adolescents with physical disabilities. *Journal of Adolescence, 34*(4), 795–80. https://doi.org/10.1016/j.adolescence.2010.04.007. Medline:20488511

Stewart, M., Castleden, H., King, M., Letourneau, N., Masuda, J., Bourque Bearskin, L., Anderson, S., & Blood, R. (2015). Supporting parents of Aboriginal children with asthma: Preferences and pilot interventions. *International Journal of Indigenous Health, 10*(2), 131–49. https://doi.org/10.3138/ijih.v10i2.29050

Stewart, M., Dennis, C-L., Kariwo, M., Kushner, K., Letourneau, N., Makumbe, M., Makwarimba, E., & Shizha, E. (2015). Challenges faced by refugee new parents from Africa in Canada. *Journal of Immigrant and Minority Health, 17*(4), 1146–56. https://doi.org/10.1007/S10903-014-0062-3. Medline:24989494

Stewart, M., Evans, J., Letourneau, N., Masuda, J., Almond, A., & Edey, J. (2016). Low-income children, adolescents, and caregivers facing respiratory problems: Support needs and preferences. *Journal of Pediatric Nursing, 31*(3), 319–29. https://doi.org/10.1016/j.pedn.2015.11.013. Medline:26968529

Stewart, M., King, M., Blood, R., Letourneau, N., Masuda, J., Anderson, S., & Bourque Bearskin, L. (2013). Health inequities experienced by

Aboriginal children with respiratory problems and their parents. *Canadian Journal of Nursing Research, 45*(3), 6–27. https://doi.org/10.1177 /084456211304500302

Stewart, M., Kushner, K.E., Dennis, C., Kariwo, M., Letourneau, N., Makumbe, K., ... Shizha, E. (2017). Social support needs of Sudanese and Zimbabwean refugee new parents in Canada. *International Journal of Migration, Health & Social Care, 13*(2), 234–52. https://doi.org/10.1108 /IJMHSC-07-2014-0028

Stewart, M., Letourneau, N., Masuda, J.R., Anderson, S., Cicuotto, L., McGhan, S.L., & Watt, S. (2012). Support needs and preferences of young adolescents with asthma and allergies: "Just no one really seems to understand." *Journal of Pediatric Nursing, 27*(5), 479–90. https://doi.org/10.1016/j.pedn.2011.06.011. Medline:22920659

Stewart, M., Letourneau, N., Masuda, J.R., Anderson, S., & McGhan, S.L. (2011). Online solutions to support needs and preferences of parents of children with asthma and allergies. *Journal of Family Nursing, 17*(3), 357–79. https://doi.org10.1177/1074840711415416

Stewart, M., Makwarimba, E., Barnfather, A., Reutter, L., Letourneau, N., & Hungler, K. (2007). Promoting the health of vulnerable populations: Collaborative research strategies. *Diversity in Health and Social Care, 4*(1), 33–48. https://pdfs.semanticscholar.org/a2f7/8e72fe136298af8a939202d9d 8d1f5fa990c.pdf

Stewart, M., Makwarimba, E., Beiser, M., Neufeld, A., Simich, P., & Spitzer, D. (2010) Social support and health: Immigrants' and refugees' perspectives. *Diversity in Health and Care, 7*(2), 91–103. http://diversityhealthcare .imedpub.com/social-support-and-health-immigrants-and-refugees-perspectives .php?aid=2006

Stewart, M., Makwarimba, E., Letourneau, N., Kushner, K., Spitzer, D., Dennis, C-L., & Shizha, E. (2015). Support intervention impacts for Zimbabwe and Sudanese refugee parents: "I am not alone." *Canadian Journal of Nursing Research, 47*(4), 113–40. https://doi.org/10.1177/084456211504700407. Medline:29509481

Stewart, M., Makwarimba, E., Reutter, L., Veenstra, G., Raphael, D., & Love, R. (2009). Poverty, sense of belonging, and experiences of social isolation. *Journal of Poverty, 13*(2), 173–95. https://doi.org/10.1080/10875540902841762

Stewart, M., Masuda, J., Evans, J., Letourneau, N., & Edey, J. (2015). Respiratory health inequities experienced by low income children and parents. *Journal of Poverty, 20*(3), 278–95. https://doi.org/10.1080/10875549 .2015.1094771

Stewart, M., Reid, G., & Mangham, C. (1997). Fostering children's resilience. *Journal of Pediatric Nursing, 12*(1), 21–31. https://doi.org/10.1016/S0882 -5963(97)80018-8

Stewart, M., Reutter, L., Makwarimba, E., Veenstra, G., Love, R., & Raphael, D. (2008). "Left out": Perspectives on social exclusion and inclusion across low-income groups. *Health Sociology Review, 17*(1), 78–94. https://doi.org/10.5172/hesr.451.17.1.78

Stewart, M., Reutter, L., Veenstra, G., Love, R., & Raphael, D. (2007). "Left out": Perspectives on social exclusion and social inclusion in low-income populations. *Canadian Journal of Nursing Research, 39*(3), 209–12. https://doi.org/10.5172/hesr.451.17.1.78. Medline:17970472

Stewart, M., Shizha, E., Makwarimba, E., Spitzer, D., Khalema, E.N., & Nsaliwa, C.D. (2011). Challenges and barriers to services for immigrant seniors in Canada: "You are among others but you feel alone." *International Journal of Migration, Health and Social Care, 7*(1), 16–32. https://doi.org/10.1108/17479891111176278

Stewart, M., Simich, L., Beiser, M., Makumbe, K., Makwarimba, E., & Shizha, E. (2011). Impacts of a social support intervention for Somali and Sudanese refugees in Canada. *Ethnicity and Inequalities in Health and Social Care, 4*(4), 186–99. https://doi.org/10.1108/17570981111250840

Stewart, M., Simich, L., Shizha, E., Makumbe, K., & Makwarimba, E. (2012). Supporting African refugees in Canada: Insights from a support intervention. *Health and Social Care in the Community, 20*(5), 516–27. https://doi.org/10.1111/j.1365-2524.2012.01069.x. Medline:22639987

Stewart, S.E., Beresin, C., Haddad, S., Egan Stack, D., Fama, J., & Jenike, M. (2008). Predictors of family accommodation in obsessive-compulsive disorder. *Annals of Clinical Psychiatry, 20*(2), 65–70. https://doi.org/10.1080/10401230802017043

Stewart, S.E., Geller, D.A., Jenike, M., Pauls, D., Shaw, D., Mullin, B., & Faraone, S.V. (2004). Long-term outcome of pediatric obsessive-compulsive disorder: a meta-analysis and qualitative review of the literature. *Acta Psychiatrica Scandinavica, 110*(1), 4–13. https://doi.org/10.1111/j.1600-0447.2004.00302.x. Medline:15180774

Stewart, S.E., Hezel, D., & Stachon, A.C. (2012). Assessment and medication management of paediatric obsessive-compulsive disorder. *Drugs, 72*(7), 881–93. https://doi.org/10.2165/11632860-000000000-00000. Medline:22564131

Stewart, S. E., Hu, Y.-P., Hezel, D. M., Proujansky, R., Lamstein, A., Walsh, C., … Pauls, D. L. (2011). Development and psychometric properties of the OCD Family Functioning (OFF) Scale. *Journal of Family Psychology, 25*(3), 434–43. https://doi.org/10.1037/a0023735. Medline:21553962

Stewart, S.E., Hu, Y.-P., Leung, A., Chan, E., Hezel, D.M., Lin, S.Y., … Pauls, D.L. (2017). A multisite study of family functioning impairment in pediatric obsessive-compulsive disorder. *Journal of the American Academy of Child & Adolescent Psychiatry, 56*(3), 241–9.e3. https://doi.org/10.1016/j.jaac.2016.12.012. Medline:28219490

Stewart, S.E., Negreiros, J., Belschner, L., & Lin, S. (2016). Neurocognition in pediatric obessive-compulsive disorder: Clinical impacts and future considerations [abstract]. Journal of the American Academy of Child & Adolescent Psychiatry, 55(10S), S291. https://doi.org/10.1016/j.jaac .2016.07.241

Stewart, S.E., Rosário, M.C., Baer, L., Carter, A.S., Brown, T.A., ... Pauls, D.L. (2008). Four-factor structure of obsessive-compulsive disorder symptoms in children, adolescents, and adults. Journal of the American Academy of Child & Adolescent Psychiatry, 47(7), 763–72. https://doi.org/10.1097/CHI .0b013e318172ef1e. Medline:18520961

Stewart, S.E., Stack, D.E., Tsilker, S., Alosso, J., Stephansky, M., Hezel, D.M., Jenike, E.A., Haddad, S.A., Kant, J., & Jenike, M.A. (2009). Long-term outcome following intensive residential treatment of obsessive-compulsive disorder. Journal of Psychiatric Research, 43(13), 1118–23. https://doi.org /10.1016/j.jpsychires.2009.03.012. Medline:19419736

Stewart, S.E., Yu, D., Scharf, J.M., Neale, B.M., Fagerness, J.A., Mathews, C.A., Arnold, P.D., ... Pauls, D.L. (2013). Genome-wide association study of obsessive-compulsive disorder. Molecular Psychiatry, 18(7), 788–98. https:// doi.org/10.1038/mp.2012.85. Medline:22889921

Storch, E.A., Bussing, R., Jacob, M.L., Nadeau, J.M., Crawford, E., Mutch, P.J., ... Murphy, T.K. (2015). Frequency and correlates of suicidal ideation in pediatric obsessive-compulsive disorder. Child Psychiatry & Human Development, 46(1), 75–83. https://doi.org/10.1007/s10578-014-0453-7. Medline:24682580

Storch, E.A., Geffken, G.R., Merlo, L.J., Jacob, M.L., Murphy, T.K., Goodman, W.K., ... Grabill, K. (2007). Family accommodation in pediatric obsessive-compulsive disorder. Journal of Clinical Child & Adolescent Psychology, 36(2), 207–16. https://doi.org/10.1080/15374410701277929. Medline:17484693

Storch, E.A., Jones, A.M., Lack, C.W., Ale, C.M., Sulkowski, M.L., Lewin, A.B., ... Murphy, T.K. (2012). Rage attacks in pediatric obsessive-compulsive disorder: phenomenology and clinical correlates. Journal of the American Academy of Child & Adolescent Psychiatry, 51(6), 582–92. https://doi.org/10.1016/j .jaac.2012.02.016. Medline:22632618

Storch, E.A., Merlo, L.J., Larson, M.J., Geffken, G.R., Lehmkuhl, H.D., Jacob, M.L., ... Goodman, W.K. (2008). Impact of comorbidity on cognitive-behavioral therapy response in pediatric obsessive-compulsive disorder. Journal of the American Academy of Child & Adolescent Psychiatry, 47(5), 583–92. https://doi.org/10.1097/CHI.0b013e31816774b1. Medline:18356759

Storch, E.A., Small, B.J., McGuire, J.F., Murphy, T.K., Wilhelm, S., & Geller, D.A. (2018). Quality of life in children and youth with obsessive-compulsive disorder. Journal of Child & Adolescent Psychopharmacology, 28(2), 104–10. https://doi.org/10.1089/cap.2017.0091. Medline:28910139

Straatmann, V.S., Lai, E., Lange, T., Campbell, M.C., Wickham, S., Andersen, A.-M. N., ... Taylor-Robinson, D. (2019). How do early-life factors explain social inequalities in adolescent mental health? Findings from the UK Millennium Cohort Study. *Journal of Epidemiology & Community Health, 73*(11), 1049–60. https://doi.org/10.1136/jech-2019-212367. Medline:31492761

Straus, S.E., Tetroe, J., & Graham, I.D. (Eds.). (2013). *Knowledge translation in health care: Moving from evidence to practice* (2nd ed.). John Wiley & Sons.

Strauss, C., Hale, L., & Stobie, B. (2015). A meta-analytic review of the relationship between family accommodation and OCD symptom severity. *Journal of Anxiety Disorders, 33*, 95–102. https://doi.org/10.1016/j.janxdis.2015.05.006. Medline:26074142

Suârez-Orozco, C., Todorova, I.L., & Louie, J. (2002). Making up for lost time: the experience of separation and reunification among immigrant families. *Family Process, 41*(4), 625–43. https://doi.org/10.1111/j.1545-5300.2002.00625.x. Medline:12613121

Subramaniam, M., Abdin, E., Vaingankar, J.A., & Chong, S.A. (2012). Obsessive-compulsive disorder: Prevalence, correlates, help-seeking and quality of life in a multiracial Asian population. *Social Psychiatry & Psychiatric Epidemiology, 47*(12), 2035–43. https://doi.org/10.1007/s00127-012-0507-8. Medline:22526825

Subramaniam, M., Soh, P., Vaingankar, J.A., Picco, L., & Chong, S. A. (2013). Quality of life in obsessive-compulsive disorder: Impact of the disorder and of treatment. *CNS Drugs, 27*(5), 367–83. https://doi.org/10.1007/s40263-013-0056-z. Medline:23580175

Suku, S., Soni, J., Martin, M.A., Mirza, M.P., Glassgow, A.E., Gerges, M., ... Caskey, R. (2019). A multivariable analysis of childhood psychosocial behaviour and household functionality. *Child Care, Health and Development, 45*(4), 551–8. https://doi.org/10.1111/cch.12665. Medline:30897231

Szaflarski, M., & Bauldry, S. (2019). The effects of perceived discrimination on immigrant and refugee physical and mental health. *Advanced Medical Sociology, 19*, 173–204. https://doi.org/10.1108/S1057-629020190000019009. Medline:31178652

Tackling the multidimensionality of child poverty. (2019). *Lancet, 3*(4), 199. https://doi.org/10.1016/S2352-4642(19)30067-7. Medline:30878106

Tafoya, T. (1982). Coyote's Eyes: Native cognition styles. *Journal of American Indian Education, 21*(2), 21–33.

Tam, T. (2019). *Addressing stigma: Towards a more inclusive health system.* Public Health Agency of Canada. www.canada.ca/en/public-health/corporate/publications/chief-public-health-officer-reports-state-public-health-canada/addressing-stigma-toward-more-inclusive-health-system.html

Taylor, M.J., Martin, J., Lu, Y., Brikell, I., Lundström, S., Larsson, H., & Lichtenstein, P. (2018). Association of genetic risk factors for psychiatric disorders and traits of these disorders in a Swedish population twin sample. *JAMA Psychiatry, 76*(3), 280–9. https://doi.org/10.1001/jamapsychiatry .2018.3652. Medline:30566181

Teixeira, C. (2008). Barriers and outcomes in the housing searches of new immigrants and refugees: A case study of "Black" Africans in Toronto's rental market. *Journal of Housing & the Built Environment, 23*(4), 253–276. https:// doi.org/10.1007/s10901-008-9118-9

Tennyson, R.D., & Volk, A. (2015). Learning theories and educational paradigm. In *International Encyclopedia of the Social & Behavioral Sciences* (2nd ed., pp. 699–711). Elsevier.

Thommasen, H.V., Baggaley, E., Thommasen, C., & Zhang, W. (2005). Prevalence of depression and prescriptions for antidepressants, Bella Coola Valley, 2001. *Canadian Journal of Psychiatry, 50*(6), 346–52. https://doi.org /10.1177/070674370505000610. Medline:15999951

Thompson-Hollands, J., Edson, A., Tompson, M.C., & Comer, J.S. (2014). Family involvement in the psychological treatment of obsessive-compulsive disorder: A meta-analysis. *Journal of Family Psychology, 28*(3), 287–98. https:// doi.org/10.1037/a0036709. Medline:24798816

Thomsen, P.H. (1995). Obsessive-compulsive disorder in children and adolescents. A 6–22 year follow-up study of social outcome. *European Child & Adolescent Psychiatry, 4*(2), 112–22. https://doi.org/10.1007/BF01977739. Medline:7796249

*Thomson, K.C., Guhn, M., Richardson, C.G., Ark, T.K., & Shoveller, J. (2017). Profiles of children's social-emotional health at school entry and associated income, gender and language inequalities: A cross-sectional population-based study in British Columbia, Canada. *BMJ Open, 7*(7), e015353. http:// dx.doi.org/10.1136/bmjopen-2016-015353

Tie, H., Krebs, G., Lang, K., Shearer, J., Turner, C., Mataix-Cols, D., Lovell, K., Heyman, I., & Byford, S. (2019). Cost-effectiveness analysis of telephone cognitive-behaviour therapy for adolescents with obsessive-compulsive disorder. *BJPsych Open, 5*(1), e7. https://doi.org/10.1192/bjo.2018.73. Medline:30762502

Tilleczek, K., Ferguson, M., Campbell, V., & Lezeu, K.E. (2014). Mental health and poverty in young lives: Intersections and directions. *Canadian Journal of Community Mental Health, 33*(1), 63–76.

Tjepkema, M., Bushnik, T., & Bougie, E. (2019). Health reports: Life expectancy of First Nations, Métis and Inuit household populations in Canada. *Statistics Canada*, Cat. No. 82.003-x. https://doi.org/10.25318 /82-003-x201901200001-eng

To, T., Dell, S., Tassoudji, M., & Wang, C. (2009). Health outcomes in low-income children with current asthma in Canada. *Chronic Diseases in Canada, 29*(2), 49–55. www.phac-aspc.gc.ca/ publicat/cdic-mcbc/29-2/pdf/cdic29-2 -3-eng.pdf

Torp, N.C., Dahl, K., Skarphedinsson, G., Compton, S., Thomsen, P.H., Weidle, B., ... Ivarsson, T. (2015). Predictors associated with improved cognitive-behavioral therapy outcome in pediatric obsessive-compulsive disorder. *Journal of the American Academy of Child & Adolescent Psychiatry, 54*(3), 200–7 e201. https://doi.org/10.1016/j.jaac.2014.12.007. Medline:25721185

Tousignant, M., Habimana, E., Biron, C., Malo, C., Sidoli-LeBlanc, E. & Bendris, N. (1999). The Quebec adolescent refugee project: Psychopathology and family variables in a sample from 35 nations. *Journal of the American Academy of Child and Adolescent Psychiatry, 38*(11), 1426–32. https://doi.org/10.1097/00004583-199911000-00018. Medline:10560230

Towle, A., Godolphin, W., & Alexander, T. (2006). Doctor-patient communications in the Aboriginal community: towards the development of educational programs. *Patient Education and Counseling, 62*(3), 340–6. https://doi.org/10.1016/j.pec.2006.06.006. Medline:16860965

Tri-Council (Canadian Institutes of Health Research, Natural Sciences and Engineering Research Council of Canada, & Social Sciences and Humanities Research Council of Canada). (2010). *Tri-Council policy statement: Ethical conduct for research involving humans.* https://ethics.gc.ca/eng/policy-politique_tcps2-eptc2_2018.html

Truth and Reconciliation Commission of Canada (TRCC). (2015). *Truth and Reconciliation Commission of Canada: Calls to action.* http://trc.ca/assets/pdf/Calls_to_Action_English2.pdf

Tsui, L., Chapman, S.A., Schnirer, L., & Stewart, S. (2006). *A handbook on knowledge sharing: Strategies and recommendations for researchers, policy makers and service providers.* Edmonton, AB: Community-University Partnership for the Study of Children, Youth, and Families. https://www.ualberta.ca/community-university-partnership/media-library/community-university-partnership/research/evaluation/knowledgesharinghandbook.pdf

Tulli, M., Salami, B., Begashaw, L., Meherali, S., Yohani, S., & Hegadoren, K. (2020). Immigrant mothers' perspectives of barriers and facilitators in accessing mental health care for their children. *Journal of Transcultural Nursing, 31*(6), 598–605. https://pubmed.ncbi.nlm.nih.gov/32013750/

Uchida, Y., Kitayama, S., Mesquita, B., Reyes, J.A.S., & Morling, B. (2008). Is perceived emotional Support beneficial? Well-being and health in independent and interdependent cultures. *Personality Social Psychology Bulletin, 34*(6), 741–54. https://doi.org/10.1177/0146167208315157. Medline:18359927

Ungar, M. 2018. Systemic resilience: Principles and processes for a science of change in contexts of adversity. *Ecology and Society, 23*(4), 34. https://doi.org/10.5751/ES-10385-230434

Ungar, M., Theron, L., Liebenberg, L., Tian, G-X., Restrepo, A., Sanders, J., Munford, R., ... Russell, S. (2015). Patterns of individual coping, engagement with social supports and use of formal services among a five-country sample of resilient youth. *Global Mental Health, 2*(e21). https://doi.org/10.1017/gmh.2015.19. Medline:28596868

Ungar, W.J., Paterson, J.M., Gomes, T., Bikangaga, P., Gold, M., To, T., & Kozyrskyj, A.L. (2011). Relationship of asthma management, socioeconomic status, and medication insurance characteristics to exacerbation frequency in children with asthma. *Annals of Allergy Asthma & Immunology, 106*(1), 17–23. https://doi.org/10.1016/j.anai.2010.10.006. Medline:21195940

UNICEF. (2009). Aboriginal children's health: Leaving no child behind. *Canadian supplement to the State of the World's Children 2009.* UNICEF Canada. https://www.unicef.ca/sites/default/files/imce_uploads/DISCOVER/OUR%20WORK/ADVOCACY/DOMESTIC/POLICY%20ADVOCACY/DOCS/Leaving%20no%20child%20behind%2009.pdf

UNICEF. (2018). *Child Migration.* https://data.unicef.org/topic/child-migration-and-displacement/migration/

United Nations (UN). (2007). *United Nations Declaration on the Rights of Indigenous Peoples.* United Nations: Department of Economic and Social Affairs- Indigenous Peoples. www.un.org/development/desa/indigenouspeoples/declaration-on-the-rights-of-indigenous-peoples.html

United Nations (UN). (2018). *International migrant stock: The 2017 revision – by destination and origin.* https://www.un.org/en/development/desa/population/migration/data/estimates2/estimates17.asp

Usman, L.M. (2012). Communication disorders and the inclusion of newcomer African refugees in rural primary schools of British Columbia, Canada. *International Journal of Progressive Education, 8*(2), 102–121.

Van Ameringen, M., Turna, J., Khalesi, Z., Pullia, K., & Patterson, B. (2017). There is an app for that! The current state of mobile applications (apps) for DSM-5 obsessive-compulsive disorder, posttraumatic stress disorder, anxiety and mood disorders. *Depression and Anxiety, 34*(6), 526–39. https://doi.org/10.1002/da.22657. Medline:28569409

Vang, Z.M., Sigouin, J., Flenon, A., & Gagnon, A. (2017). Are immigrants healthier than native-born Canadians? A systematic review of the healthy immigrant effect in Canada. *Ethnicity & Health, 22*(3), 209–41. https://doi.org/10.1080/13557858.2016.1246518. Medline:27809589

Van Herk, K.A., Smith, D., & Andrew, C. (2011). Identity matters: Aboriginal mothers' experiences of accessing health care. *Contemporary Nurse, 37*(1), 57–68. https://doi.org/10.5172/conu.2011.37.1.057. Medline:21591827

Varcoe, C., Browne, A., & Garneau, A.B. (2019). Beyond stress and coping: The relevance of critical theoretical perspectives to conceptualising racial discrimination in health research. *Health Sociology Review, 28*(3), 245–60. https://doi.org/10.1080/14461242.2019.1642124

Vaughn, L.M., Wagner, E., & Jacquez, F. (2013). A review of community-based participatory research in child health. *The American Journal of Maternal Child Nursing, 38*(1), 48–53. https://doi.org/10.1097/NMC.0b013e31826591a3. Medline:23232779

Velloso, P., Piccinato, C., Ferrão, Y., Perin, E.A., Cesar, R., Fontenelle, L.F., Hounie, A.G., & do Rosário, M.C. (2018). Clinical predictors of quality of life in a large sample of adult obsessive-compulsive disorder outpatients. *Comprehensive Psychiatry, 86*, 82–90. https://doi.org/10.1016/j.comppsych .2018.07.007. Medline:30086510

Venables, R.W. (2008). *Polishing the Silver Covenant Chain: A brief history of some of the symbols and metaphors in Haudenosaunee treaty negotiations.* Onandaga Nation: People of the Hills. http://honorthetworow.org/wp-content /uploads/2013/03/Venables-on-the-Covenant-Chain-of-Treaties.pdf

Victorino, C.C., & Gauthier, A.H. (2009). The social determinants of child health: Variations across health outcomes – A population-based cross-sectional analysis. *BMC Pediatrics, 9*, 53–64. https://doi.org/10.1186/1471 -2431-9-53. Medline:19686599

Vikas, A., Avasthi, A., & Sharan, P. (2011). Psychosocial impact of obsessive-compulsive disorder on patients and their caregivers: A comparative study with depressive disorder. *International Journal of Social Psychiatry, 57*(1), 45–56. https://doi.org/10.1177/0020764010347333. Medline:21252355

Visser, H.A., van Minnen, A., van Megen, H., Eikelenboom, M., Hoogendoorn, A.W., Kaarsemaker, M., ... van Oppen, P. (2014). The relationship between adverse childhood experiences and symptom severity, chronicity, and comorbidity in patients with obsessive-compulsive disorder. *Journal of Clinical Psychiatry, 75*(10), 1034–9. https://doi.org/10.4088/JCP.13m08825. Medline:25006863

Vonneilich, N., Lüdecke, D., & Kofahl, C. (2016). The impact of care on family and health-related quality of life of parents with chronically ill and disabled children. *Disability and Rehabilitation, 38*(8), 761–7. https://doi.org/10.3109 /09638288.2015.1060267

von Rueden, U., Gosch, A., Rajmil, L., Bisegger, C., & Ravens-Sieberer, U. (2006). Socioeconomic determinants of health related quality of life in childhood and adolescence: Results from a European study. *Journal of Epidemiology & Community Health, 60*(2), 130–5. https://doi.org/10.1136 /jech.2005.039792. Medline:16415261

Waddell, C., Georgiades, K., Duncan, L., Comeau, J., Reid, G.J., O'Briain, W., ... Ontario Child Health Study Team. (2019). 2014 Ontario Child Health Study findings: Policy implications for Canada. *Canadian Journal of Psychiatry, 64*(4), 227–31. https://doi.org/10.1177/0706743719830033. Medline:30978136

Waddell, C., Offord, D.R., Shepherd, C.A., Hua, J.M., & McEwan, K. (2002). Child psychiatric epidemiology and Canadian public policy-making:

The state of the science and the art of the possible. *Canadian Journal of Psychiatry, 47*(9), 825–32. https://doi.org/10.1177/070674370204700903. Medline:12500752

Wang, J.J., Lin, S., Best, J.R., Selles, R.R., & Stewart, S.E. (2020). Race and ethnicity in pediatric OCD: An exploratory study of a clinical North American sample. *Annals of Clinical Psychiatry, 32*(4), e2–15.

Warner, F.R. (2007). Social support and distress among Q'eqchi refugee woman in Maya Tecun, Mexico. *Medical Anthropology Quarterly, 21*(2), 193–217. https://doi.org/10.1525/maq.2007.21.2.193. Medline:17601084

Waters, T.L., & Barrett, P.M. (2000). The role of the family in childhood obsessive-compulsive disorder. *Clinical Child & Family Psychology Reviews, 3*(3), 173–84. https://doi.org/10.1023/a:1009551325629. Medline:11225752

Watson, H.J., & Rees, C.S. (2008). Meta-analysis of randomized, controlled treatment trials for pediatric obsessive-compulsive disorder. *Journal of Child Psychology & Psychiatry, 49*(5), 489–98. https://doi.org/10.1111/j.1469 -7610.2007.01875.x. Medline:18400058

Weinert, C. (2003). Measuring social support: PRQ2000. In O. Strickland and C. Dilorio (Eds.), *Measurement of nursing outcomes: Self care and coping* (2nd ed., pp. 161–72). New York, NY: Springer.

Weiss, H.A., & Ferrand, R.A. (2019). Improving adolescent health: An evidence-based call to action. *The Lancet, 393*(10176), 1073–5. https://doi.org/10.1016 /S0140-6736(18)32996-9. Medline:30876704

Weissman, M.M., Bland, R.C., Canino, G.J., Greenwald, S., Hwu, H.G., Lee, C.K., Newman, S.C., Oakley-Browne, M.A., Rubio-Stipec, M., Wickramaratne, P.J., & et al. (1994). The cross national epidemiology of obsessive compulsive disorder. The Cross National Collaborative Group. *Journal of Clinical Psychiatry, 55*(Suppl.), 5–10. Medline:8077177

Wellen, B., Skriner, L.C., Freeman, J., Stewart, E., Garcia, A., Sapyta, J., & Franklin, M. (2017). Examining the psychometric properties of the Pediatric Quality of Life Enjoyment and Satisfaction Questionnaire in two samples of youth with OCD. *Child Psychiatry & Human Development, 48*(1), 180–8. https://doi.org/10.1007/s10578-016-0662-3. Medline: 27329368

Wendt, D.C., Hartmann, W.E., Allen, J., Burack, J.A., Charles, B., D'Amico, E.J., … Walls, M.L. (2019). Substance use research with Indigenous communities: Exploring and extending foundational principles of community psychology. *American Journal of Community Psychology, 64*(1–2), 146–58. https://doi.org /10.1002/ajcp.12363. Medline:31365138

Westwell-Roper, C., & Stewart, S.E. (2019). Challenges in the diagnosis and treatment of pediatric obsessive-compulsive disorder. *Indian Journal of Psychiatry, 61*(Suppl. 1), S119–S130. https://doi.org/10.4103/psychiatry. IndianJPsychiatry_524_18. Medline:30745685

Westwell-Roper, C., Williams, K.A., Samuels, J., Bienvenu, O.J., Cullen, B., Goes, F.S., ... Stewart, S.E. (2019). Immune-related comorbidities in childhood-onset obsessive compulsive disorder: Lifetime prevalence in the Obsessive Compulsive Disorder Collaborative Genetics Association Study. *Journal of Child & Adolescent Psychopharmacology, 29*(8). https://doi.org/10.1089/cap .2018.0140. Medline:31170001

Wetterneck, C.T., Little, T.E., Rinehart, K.L., Cervantes, M.E., Hyde, E., & Williams, M. (2012). Latinos with obsessive-compulsive disorder: Mental healthcare utilization and inclusion in clinical trials. *Journal of Obsessive-Compulsive and Related Disorders, 1*(2), 85–97. https://doi.org/10.1016 /j.jocrd.2011.12.001. Medline:29057210

Wexler, L.M., DiFluvio, G., & Burke, T.K. (2009). Resilience and marginalized youth: Making a case for personal and collective meaning-making as part of resilience research in public health. *Social Science & Medicine, 69*(4), 565–70. https://doi.org/10.1016/j.socscimed.2009.06.022. Medline:19596503

Whitaker, A., Johnson, J., Shaffer, D., Rapoport, J.L., Kalikow, K., Walsh, B.T., ... Dolinsky, A. (1990). Uncommon troubles in young people: Prevalence estimates of selected psychiatric disorders in a nonreferred adolescent population. *Archives of General Psychiatry, 47*(5), 487–96. https://doi .org/10.1001/archpsyc.1990.01810170087013. Medline:2331210

Whitbeck, L.B., Yu, M., Johnson, K.D., Hoyt, D.R., & Walls, M.L. (2008). Diagnostic prevalence rates from early to mid-adolescence among indigenous adolescents: First results from a longitudinal study. *Journal of the American Academy of Child & Adolescent Psychiatry, 47*(8), 890–900. https://doi .org/10.1097/CHI.0b013e3181799609. Medline:18596558

Wiik, K.L., Loman, M.M., Van Ryzin, M.J., Armstrong, J.M., Essex, M.J., Pollak, S.D., & Gunnar, M.R. (2011). Behavioral and emotional symptoms of post-institutionalized children in middle childhood. *Journal of Child Psychology & Psychiatry, 52*(1), 56–63. https://doi.org/10.1111/j.1469-7610.2010.02294.x. Medline:20649913

Wille, N., Bettge, S., Ravens-Sieberer, U., & BELLA Study Group. (2008). Risk and protective factors for children's and adolescents' mental health: results of the BELLA study. *European Child & Adolescent Psychiatry, 17*(1), 133–47. https://doi.org/10.1007/s00787-008-1015-y. Medline:19132313

Williams, D.R., & Cooper, L.A. (2019). Reducing racial inequities in health: Using what we already know to take action. *International Journal of Environmental Research and Public Health, 16*(4). https://doi.org/10.3390 /ijerph16040606. Medline:30791452

Williams, D.R., Lawrence, J.A., & Davis, B.A. (2019). Racism and health: Evidence and needed research. *Annual Review of Public Health, 40*, 105–25. https://www.annualreviews.org/doi/pdf/10.1146/annurev-publhealth -040218-043750

Williams, D.R., & Mohammed, S.A. (2013). Racism and health II: A needed research agenda for effective interventions. *American Behavioral Scientist, 57*(8), 1200–26. https://doi.org/10.1177/0002764213487341. Medline:24347667

Williams, D.R., Priest, N., & Anderson N.B. (2016). Understanding associations among race, socioeconomic status, and health: Patterns and prospects. *Health Psychology, 35*(4), 407–11. https://doi.org/1037/hea0000242. Medline:27018733

Williams, M.T., Domanico, J., Marques, L., Leblanc, N.J., & Turkheimer, E. (2012). Barriers to treatment among African Americans with obsessive-compulsive disorder. *Journal of Anxiety Disorders, 26*(4), 555–63. https://doi.org/10.1016/j.janxdis.2012.02.009. Medline:22410094

Williams, M.T., Elstein, J., Buckner, E., Abelson, J., & Himle, J. (2012). Symptom dimensions in two samples of Africans Americans with obsessive-compulsive disorder. *Journal of Obsessive-Compulsive Related Disorders, 1*(3), 145–52. https://doi.org/10.1016/j.jocrd.2012.03.004. Medline:22708117

Williams, M.T., & Jahn, M.E. (2017). Obsessive-compulsive disorder in African American children and adolescents: Risks, resiliency, and barriers to treatment. *American Journal of Orthopsychiatry, 87*(3), 291–303. https://doi.org/10.1037/ort0000188. Medline:27243576

Williams, M.T., Powers, M., Yun, Y.-G., & Foa, E. (2010). Minority participation in randomized controlled trials for obsessive-compulsive disorder. *Journal of Anxiety Disorders, 24*(2), 171–7. https://doi.org/10.1016/j.janxdis.2009.11.004. Medline:20143498

Williams, M.T., Taylor, R.J., Himle, J.A., & Chatters, L.M. (2017). Demographic and health-related correlates of obsessive-compulsive symptoms among African Americans. *Journal of Obsessive-Compulsive Related Disorders, 14*, 119–26. https://doi.org/10.1016/j.jocrd.2017.07.001. Medline:30079297

Witthauer, C., Gloster, A.T., Meyer, A.H., & Lieb, R. (2014). Physical diseases among persons with obsessive compulsive symptoms and disorder: a general population study. *Social Psychiatry and Psychiatric Epidemiology, 49*(12), 2013–22. https://doi.org/10.1007/s00127-014-0895-z. Medline:24907897

Woodgate, R.L., & Busolo, D.S. (2018). Above chaos, quest, and restitution: Narrative experiences of African immigrant youth's settlement in Canada. *BMC Public Health, 18*(1), 333. https://doi.org/10.1186/s12889-018-5239-6. Medline:29514615

World Health Organization (WHO). (2014). *Health for the world's adolescents: A second chance in the second decade.* https://www.who.int/maternal_child_adolescent/topics/adolescence/second-decade/en/

World Health Organization (WHO). (2018). *Key learning on health in all policies implementation from around the world.*https://apps.who.int/iris/bitstream/handle/10665/272711/WHO-CED-PHE-SDH-18.1-eng.pdf

World Health Organization (WHO). (2019). *About social determinants of health.* www.who.int/social_determinants/sdh_definition/en/

World Health Organization and the Calouste Gulbenkian Foundation (WHO & CGF). (2014). *Social determinants of mental health.* https://www.who .int/mental_health/publications/gulbenkian_paper_social_determinants_of _mental_health/en/

Wright, A.L., Jack, S.M., Ballantyne, M., Gabel, C., Bomberry, R., & Wahoush, O. (2019). How Indigenous mothers experience selecting and using early childhood development services to care for their infants. *International Journal of Qualitative Studies on Health and Wellbeing, 14*(1). https://doi.org/10.1080 /17482631.2019.1601486. Medline:30982415

Wu, M.S., Geller, D.A., Schneider, S.C., Small, B.J., Murphy, T.K., Wilhelm, S., & Storch, E.A. (2019). Comorbid psychopathology and the clinical profile of family accommodation in pediatric OCD. *Child Psychiatry & Human Development, 26*, 624. https://doi.org/10.1007/s10578-019-00876-7. Medline:30790098

Wu, M.S., Pinto, A., Horng, B., Phares, V., McGuire, J.F., Dedrick, R.F., ... Storch, E.A. (2016). Psychometric properties of the Family Accommodation Scale for Obsessive-Compulsive Disorder-Patient Version. *Psychological Assessment, 28*(3), 251–62. https://doi.org/10.1037/pas0000165. Medline:26075408

Yang, C., Nestadt, G., Samuels, J.F., & Doerfler, L.A. (2018). Cross-cultural differences in the perception and understanding of obsessive-compulsive disorder in East Asian and Western cultures. *International Journal of Culture & Mental Health, 11*(4), 616–25. https://doi.org/10.1080/17542863.2018 .1468786

Yorulmaz, O., Gençöz, T., & Woody, S. (2010). Vulnerability factors in OCD symptoms: Cross-cultural comparisons between Turkish and Canadian samples. *Clinical Psychology & Psychotherapy, 17*(2), 110–21. https://doi.org /10.1002/cpp.642. Medline:19701960

Young, C., Hanson, C., Craig, J.C., Clapham, K., & Williamson, A. (2017). Psychosocial factors associated with the mental health of indigenous children living in high income countries: A systematic review. *International Journal of Equity in Health, 16*(1), 153. https://doi.org/10.1186/s12939-017-0652-5. Medline:28830449

Zaboski, B.A., Gilbert, A., Hamblin, R., Andrews, J., Ramos, A., Nadeau, J.M., & Storch, E.A. (2019). Quality of life in children and adolescents with obsessive-compulsive disorder: The Pediatric Quality of Life Enjoyment and Satisfaction Questionnaire (PQ-LES-Q). *Bulletin of the Menninger Clinic*, 1–21. https://doi.org/10.1521/bumc_2019_83_03. Medline:31180235

Zilanawala, A., Sacker, A., & Kelly, Y. (2019). Internalising and externalising behaviour profiles across childhood: The consequences of changes in the

family environment. *Social Science & Medicine, 226*, 207–16. https://doi
.org/10.1016/j.socscimed.2019.02.048. Medline:30870739

Zimet, G.D., Dahlem, N.W., Zimet, S.G., & Farley, G.K. (1988). The
Multidimensional Scale of Perceived Social Support. *Journal of Personality
Assessment, 52*(1): 30–41. https://doi.org/10.1207/s15327752jpa5201_2

Contributors

Dominic A. Alaazi, PhD, is a postdoctoral fellow at the College of Health Sciences, University of Alberta. He holds a PhD in Public Health from the University of Alberta and has previously worked as a research coordinator for the Health and Immigration Policies and Practices Research Program (HIPP), where he supported the implementation of funded projects on the health and well-being of immigrant populations in Alberta and across Canada. He also received an MPhil degree in Environmental Science from the University of Ghana and an MA in Human Geography from the University of Manitoba.

Sharon Anderson received her PhD from the Department of Human Ecology, University of Alberta, obtained a Master of Science in Health Promotion at the University of Alberta, and a Master of Education in Community Rehabilitation and Disability Studies at the University of Calgary. She is the recipient of fifteen academic awards, including the Dorothy J. Killam Memorial Doctoral Graduate Prize, the Izaak Walton Killam Memorial Doctoral Scholarships, the Social Sciences and Humanities Doctoral Fellowship, two Queen Elizabeth II Graduate Scholarships, and the Andrew Stewart Memorial Graduate Scholarship. She has twenty-three papers published in peer-reviewed journals. She enhanced her knowledge of social support and participatory community-engaged research as a research assistant and then as a research associate in the Social Support Research Program led by Dr. Miriam Stewart at the University of Alberta. The opportunity to work with Indigenous children and their parents was a highlight of her work in this research program. It enabled her to reconnect with her paternal great-grandmother's roots. She currently works as a research coordinator for Dr. Jasneet Parmar at the University of Alberta and the Network of Excellence in Seniors Health and Wellness.

R. **Lisa Bourque Bearskin**, PhD, is a member of Beaver Lake Cree Nation in Treaty 6 Territory, and an associate professor and New Researcher in the School of Nursing at Thompson Rivers University. She is affiliated with the Canadian Association of Schools of Nursing, the International Public Health Association, and the Canadian Indigenous Nurses Association. As past president of CINA, she contributed to the advancement of Indigenous-nursing leadership. She has worked in community health at the Maskwacis Community College/Health Centre in Alberta; at the Arctic Nursing program in Iqaluit Nunavut; and at the University of Alberta's Faculty of Nursing where she developed and delivered Indigenous-nursing initiatives. She was awarded her PhD in Nursing in 2014. In 2017, she received the Canadian Nurses Association Award for the Top 150 Nurses. She most recently worked on projects funded by the CIHR Institute of Indigenous Peoples Health. Her research focuses on addressing Indigenous health inequities by supporting Indigenous wellness research led by Indigenous communities. She is working with nurses and various communities to enhance understandings of Indigenous nursing knowledge and social determinants of health, which maintains cultural integrity of nurses' practice and supports Indigenous clients' security and sovereignty.

Jocelyn Edey, MSc, is a research assistant in the Faculty of Nursing at the University of Alberta. She works with Dr. Miriam Stewart in designing and implementing successful research proposals and projects, and is the co-author of published articles in a variety of journals (e.g., *International Journal of Migration, Health and Social Care, Journal of Pediatric Nursing, Journal of Poverty, The California Reader*). After receiving a Master of Science in Health Promotion from the University of Alberta, she worked for twenty years as a community development coordinator/researcher, policy analyst, academic coordinator, and researcher at the University of Calgary, University of Alberta, and University of California, Riverside. Her research interests include adolescent stress, coping, and identity; support-education intervention programs for at-risk populations; and refugee adolescent and new parent support interventions.

Carla Hilario, PhD, is an assistant professor in the Faculty of Nursing at the University of Alberta. Her research program focuses on health equity and mental health promotion with vulnerable youth. Her doctoral work examined the social context of mental health from the perspectives of immigrant and refugee young men. She is currently leading a multisite study exploring stakeholder perspectives on mental health of newcomer young men. She was recently awarded a Social Sciences and Humanities

Research Council of Canada Insight Development Grant focused on engaging Indigenous and newcomer youth in contributing to the Truth and Reconciliation Commission's Calls to Action in Canada.

Alexandra King, MD, is a member of the Nipissing First Nation (Ontario). She is an Internal Medicine Specialist with a focus on HIV/AIDS, hepatitis C (HCV), and HIV/HCV co-infections. She is the inaugural Cameco Chair in Indigenous Health and Wellness at the University of Saskatchewan. She is working with Indigenous communities and relevant stakeholders to understand the health needs of First Nations and Métis peoples in Saskatchewan, and the structural changes that are needed for improved Indigenous health outcomes. She leads work to enhance Indigenous health education; advocates for improvements and funding; ensures sustainability of effective services and supports; and facilitates knowledge and resource mobilization to support improved Indigenous health and wellness. As a First Nation researcher, she is a Principal Investigator on various CIHR research grants related to Indigenous people and HIV, HCV, and HIV/HCV co-infections.

Malcolm King, PhD, FCAHS, is a member of the Mississaugas of the New Credit First Nation, and is the Scientific Director of the Saskatchewan Centre for Patient-Oriented Research. He also served as Scientific Director of CIHR's Institute of Aboriginal Peoples' Health. He was a professor at the University of Alberta and an Alberta Heritage Foundation for Medical Research Senior Scholar in Pulmonary Medicine. At Simon Fraser University, he co-led the development of an Indigenous Health in Canada course. His academic interests include health issues experienced by Indigenous peoples, health service delivery to vulnerable populations, and the interaction of education and health. He is the author of approximately 200 scientific papers. He was honoured with a National Aboriginal Achievement Award in 1999, and, in 2016, he was named a Fellow of the Canadian Academy of Health Sciences.

Nicole Letourneau, PhD, RN, FCAHS, FAAN, holds the Alberta Children's Hospital Foundation Research Chair in Parent-Infant Mental Health and is director of RESOLVE Alberta (focused on family violence research and education). Formerly, she was a Canada Research Chair in Healthy Child Development. Her Child Health Intervention and Longitudinal Development Studies Program tests interventions that support the development of children in families affected by toxic stressors, including parental depression and low-income. Much of her research comes from her work as Principal Investigator of the APrON longitudinal cohort study of parents and children followed since pregnancy. She is also Principal Investigator of the ATTACH™ and VID-KIDS intervention programs, designed to help parents affected by toxic stress (e.g., mental health issues, family violence, addictions, low income) nurture their children's behavioural and cognitive development and health. Her research program aims to improve development and health outcomes for at-risk children via support interventions. She has published three books – *What Kind of Parent Am I? Self-Surveys that Reveal the Impact of Toxic Stress and More* (2018); *Scientific Parenting: What Science Reveals about Parental Influence* (2013); and *Parenting and Child Development: Issues and Answers* (2020) – forty-three book chapters, and nearly 200 peer-reviewed articles and has given more than 300 presentations.

Bukola Salami, PhD, is an associate professor at the Faculty of Nursing, University of Alberta. She is the principal investigator and lead on the Health and Immigration Policies and Practices Research Program. Over the last seven years, she has been engaged in around sixty funded research studies on immigrant health. One major theme of her research program is immigrant children's mental health. Her research has been funded by provincial, national, and international funding agencies, including the Social Sciences and Humanities Research Council of Canada, the Worldwide Universities Network, Policy Wise for Children and Families, MSI Foundation, and Women and Children's Health Research Institute. She is a member of the Public Health Agency of Canada Mental Health of Black Canadian working group and she represents the University of Alberta on the steering committee of the Worldwide Universities Network Global Africa Group. She led a Worldwide Universities Network funded project with twenty scholars from four continents and nine countries on a review of the global literature on African child health. She is the founder of Africa Child and Youth Migration Network, a network of thirty-two researchers across the globe. She has received several awards in recognition of her research excellence, including the College and Association of Registered Nurses of Alberta Excellence Award, the Sigma Theta Tau International Honor Society of Nursing Excellence Award, and Edmonton's Top 40 Under 40.

Miriam J. Stewart, PhD, FRSC, FCAHS, held many leadership positions prior to her current role as Professor Emeritus, including Director and Chair of the Centre for Health Promotion Studies, University of Alberta; Director of the Atlantic Health Promotion Research Centre; co-principal investigator of the Maritime Centre of Excellence on Women's Health; and inaugural Scientific Director of the Institute of Gender and Health at the Canadian Institutes of Health Research. She successfully secured over 130 research grants from national agencies (e.g., Canadian Institutes of Health Research, Social Sciences and Humanities Research Council of Canada), and designed and tested innovative interventions tailored to improving the lives of vulnerable Canadians across the lifespan. She has delivered over 500 presentations at national and international professional and academic conferences, and has published extensively, writing over 150 peer-reviewed articles in numerous academic and professional journals (e.g., *Social Science and Medicine, Diversity in Health and Care, Global Health Promotion, International Journal of Indigenous Health, Journal of Adolescent Health, Issues in Comprehensive Pediatric Nursing, International Journal of Nursing Studies*). She has written thirty-one book chapters and five preceding books: *Chronic Conditions and Caregiving in Canada: Social Support Strategies* (2000); *Community Nursing: Promoting Canadians' Health* (2000); *Community Nursing: Promoting Canadians' Health* (1995); *Integrating Social Support in Nursing* (1993); and *Community Health Nursing in Canada* (1985). Key awards include the Alberta Heritage Foundation for Medical Research Health Senior Investigator; the Alberta Heritage Foundation for Medical Research Health Senior Scholar; the, Medical Research Council of Canada and National Health Research Development Program Scholar; the Kaplan Award for Excellence in Research; and the Centennial Medal by Canadian Nurses Association of Canada. She is a Fellow of the Royal Society of Canada and a Fellow of the Canadian Academy of Health Sciences; a member of the McMaster University Alumni Gallery; and is included in *Who's Who in Canada* and *Who's Who in America.*

S. Evelyn Stewart, MD, FRCPS, is a professor in the Department of Psychiatry, University of British Columbia, and is founding medical director of the BC Children's Hospital Provincial Obsessive-Compulsive Disorder Program. She is Research Lead for Brain, Behaviour, and Development at BC Children's Hospital Research Institute, and Research Director for BC Children's Hospital Child, Youth, and Reproductive Mental Health. She has published over 100 peer-reviewed papers, meta-analyses, and chapters on origins, clinical implications, and treatment of obsessive-compulsive disorder and related mental health conditions. In 2018, she received one of the two annual UBC Faculty of Medicine Distinguished Achievement Awards for Excellence in recognition of significant and outstanding contributions to clinical and applied research. She has received numerous awards and research grants from international, national, and provincial organizations. Her current research is aimed at identifying clinical markers to improve long-term outcomes via resilience optimizing

interventions and treatment strategies for vulnerable children and adolescents. These current and ongoing clinical, family-based, genetic, imag-
ing, and cognition studies focus on OCD-affected and at-risk siblings,
and their long-term outcomes. She has been inspired throughout her
own life by the resilience, dedication, and unprecedented achievements
of her mother, Dr. Miriam Stewart.

Clara Westwell-Roper, MD, PhD, is a psychiatry research resident in the
Faculty of Medicine at the University of British Columbia. She completed
medical school with top standing in her graduating class and received a
Vanier Canada Graduate Scholarship (Canada's most prestigious graduate award recognizing academic and leadership potential) during her
PhD training. As an early career MD/PhD clinician-scientist, her research
goals are to understand better how stress and the immune system interact
to affect the developing brain. In the past ten years, she has published
twenty peer-reviewed articles, in addition to more than fifteen peer-
reviewed abstracts, and has presented twenty talks at national and international meetings. Her recent work under the mentorship of Dr. Evelyn
Stewart includes characterization of immune-related co-morbidities in
childhood-onset OCD. She is the recipient of a 2019 Young Investigator
Award from the International OCD Foundation.

Index

Page numbers in *italics* refer to figures and tables.

Aboriginal Capacity and Developmental Research Environments, 147

Aboriginal Children's Survey, 32

Aboriginal peoples, use of term, 3n1. *See also* Indigenous peoples

academic skills, and obsessive-compulsive disorder (OCD), 51–2

accessibility, 162. *See also* online support programs

adolescents, 81–2. *See also* Indigenous adolescents; low-income adolescents, with respiratory challenges; mental health, adolescents and children; Syrian refugee adolescents

adverse childhood experiences: mental health and, 31; obsessive-compulsive disorder and, 43, *48*

African immigrant children, and mental health: about, 8, 11, 16, 66, 69; pre-emigration traumas, 69–70, 75; research, practice, and policy implications, 75–7; service utilization, 74–5; sociocultural determinants of, 72–4; structural determinants of, 70–2

African immigrants, use of term, 66n1. *See also* refugee new parents

allergies, 17, 136. *See also* Indigenous children, with respiratory challenges; low-income adolescents, with respiratory challenges

Allergy and Anaphylaxis Australia, 163

Allergy Pals/Allergy Allies program, 163

Anaphylaxis Canada (now Food Allergy Canada), 157, 163

anxiety disorders, 33, 34, 41–2, 50, 59

apps, mental health, 63

asthma, 17, 92, 125, 127, 136. *See also* Indigenous children, with respiratory challenges; low-income adolescents, with respiratory challenges

Asthma Society of Canada, 163

At Home/Chez Soi study, 32

Attachment and Child Health (ATTACH™) program, 153–4, 156, 158–9

attention deficit hyperactivity disorder (ADHD), 30, 50

Australia, 163

Barriers to Treatment Participation
   Scale, 59
Barriers to Treatment Questionnaire, 59
BC Children's Hospital Provincial
   OCD Program, 61
Black Canadians, use of term,
   66n1. *See also* African immigrant
   children, and mental health;
   refugee new parents
blood-borne infections, 92, 99
Brokenleg, Martin, 98

Camp Blue Spruce, 163
Canada Health Act, 125
Canadian Community Health Survey
   (CCHS), 30, 34, 42, 59, 67
Canadian Health Measures Survey, 68
Canadian Institute for Obsessive
   Compulsive Disorders
   Accreditation Task Force, 63
Canadian Institutes of Health
   Research (CIHR), 95, 96, 147
Canadian Medical Association
   (CMA), 6
Canadian Mental Health Survey, 67
capacity building, 10
caregivers, 121–2. *See also* families;
   Indigenous parents and caregivers;
   knowledge translation; low-income
   parents and caregivers; postpartum
   depression; refugee new parents
CheckUp project, 99–100
Chief Public Health Officer: *Report on
   the State of Public Health in Canada*,
   8, 61
childcare, 126, 132, 134, 142
Child Health Study, 60
children, 15–16. *See also* African
   immigrant children, and mental
   health; Indigenous children, with
   respiratory challenges; mental
   health, adolescents and children

child welfare system, 72, 76
Circle of Courage, 98
clomipramine, 56
cognitive behavioural therapy, 54, 56,
   57, 62–3
collaboration, interdisciplinary, 12,
   164–5, 166
colonialism, 35, 36, 92, 98
Commission on Social Determinants
   of Health (CSDH), 8
communication, 131
community-based participatory
   research, 9, 10, 137, 151
community outreach, 132
community psychology, 36
computer skills, 104, 115–16, 128.
   See also online support programs;
   social media
conduct disorder, 30, 35
Cooper, L.A., 27
coping strategies, 115, 129–30, 162
COVID-19 pandemic, 63, 65
Coyote's Eyes, 95
culture: African immigrants and,
   72–3; childhood-onset mental
   health and, 61; as health
   determinant, 7–8; Indigenous
   children with respiratory
   challenges and, 21, 22, 139;
   mental health service utilization
   and, 74–5; multiculturalism, 107;
   obsessive-compulsive disorder
   and, 39–40, *48*

Dakota Tipi First Nation, 138, 143
depression, 32, 33, 34, 41–2, 67, 69.
   See also major depressive disorder;
   postpartum depression
diabetes, type 2, 92, 98
discrimination: employment and
   wage, 71; health care, 127. *See also*
   racism

domestic (intimate partner) violence, 31, 152, 153

Eczema Society of Canada, 163
education system, 22–3, 71, 73–4, 107
emotional abuse, 31
employment discrimination, 71
enuresis, 50
environmental health risks, 17, 23, 31, 36–7, 127, 139
Ermine, Willie, 93
Ethical Space, 93–4, *94*
ethnicity: definition, 39; future directions and, 165–6, 167; as health determinant, 7–8, 163–5; mental health and, 68, 76; obsessive-compulsive disorder and, 39–40, *48*, 58–9; support interventions and, 160
Etuaptmumk (Two-eyed Seeing), 9, 94–5, *95*, 160

families: African immigrants and, 72–3; death of family member, 31; Indigenous families, 135; obsessive-compulsive disorder and, *49*, 52–5; single-parent families, 34, 123
First Nations. *See* Indigenous peoples
First Nations Child and Family Service program, 137
First Nations Mental Wellness Continuum, 36
First Nations Regional Health Survey, 42
Food Allergy Canada (formerly Anaphylaxis Canada), 157, 163
food insecurity, 33, 50, 61

gender: adverse childhood experiences and, 43; CheckUp project and, 99; future directions and, 167; mental health programs and, 76; obsessive-compulsive disorder and, *47*
gender-related minority youth, 36
genetic counselling, 55
geography and rural residence: accessibility considerations, 88, 162; as health determinant, 92; Indigenous peoples and, 22, 26, 139, 140; mental health in children and, 32–3; obsessive-compulsive disorder and, 39, *47*, *48*, 53

health care: discrimination in, 127; engagement with Indigenous peoples, 144–7, 148–9. *See also* service providers
health inequalities: approach to, 4–5, 11–12, 167; ethnicity and cultural determinants, 7–8; future research and program directions, 165–7; income determinants, 5–6; methodological approaches and, 9–11; research gaps, 3–4; social support determinants, 8–9; theoretical foundations of book, 5. *See also* adolescents; children; parents; research methodologies; social determinants of health
healthy immigrant effect, 67
homelessness, 32, 36, 72
housing: African immigrants and, 71–2, 76; low-income parents and, 125, 127; mental health in children and, 32; respiratory challenges and, 23, 86, 139

immigrants: in Canada, 66; definition, 3n2; healthy immigrant effect, 67; marginalization of, 7; mental health and, 15, 33–5, 67–9. *See also* African immigrant

immigrants (*cont'd*)
  children, and mental health;
  refugees
income and poverty: financial stress,
  125–6, 159; as health determinant,
  5–6, 123–4, 163–5; low income, 83,
  123–4; mental health in children
  and, 30–1; obsessive-compulsive
  disorder and, *47*, 50; respiratory
  challenges and, 18, 23, 91; social
  support and, 8, 161. *See also*
  low-income adolescents, with
  respiratory challenges; low-income
  parents and caregivers
Indigenous adolescents: about, 11,
  81–2, 92–3, 100, 136; CheckUp
  project and sexually transmitted
  and blood-borne diseases, 99–100;
  common health issues, 92;
  Indigenous Youth Mentorship
  Program and diabetes, 98–9, 99–100;
  mental health and, 35–6, 61, 92
Indigenous children, with respiratory
  challenges: about, 7, 11, 15, 28,
  136; culture and, 21, 22, 139;
  environmental factors, 17, 23;
  hospitalization rates, 18; income
  and, 18, 23; intersectionality
  and, 26; isolation and, 21–2;
  lack of knowledge and, 22;
  methodological approach, 19–21;
  racism and, 19, 22–3, 27; risk
  factors, 18–19; smoking and, 23;
  stigma, stereotypes, and exclusion,
  21; support interventions, 23–6,
  26–7; treatment issues, 18
Indigenous parents and caregivers:
  about, 12, 121–2, 136–7; culturally
  responsive approaches, 137–8;
  engagement by service providers,
  144–7, 148–9; knowledge
  translation and, 152–3;

methodological approach, 138–9;
  research insights and implications,
  147–9; support interventions,
  142–4, 147–8, 162; support needs
  and intervention preferences,
  139–42, 161
Indigenous peoples: about, 159;
  asthma and allergies among, 17,
  136; collaboration with, 164, 166;
  Elders, 22, 93, 97, 98, 99, 138,
  140, 142; Ethical Space, 93–4,
  94; families, 135; foundational
  principles when working
  with, 9, 93–7, 100; health care
  engagement with, 144–7, 148–9;
  health inequalities, 136; low
  income and, 123; mental health
  in children and youth, 35–6, 61;
  obsessive-compulsive disorder
  in, 41–2; population, 135; social
  determinants of health for, 36, 92;
  strengths-based approaches, 95–7,
  97, 164; suicide among youth, 49;
  trauma from colonialism, 35, 98;
  Two-eyed Seeing (*Etuaptmumk*),
  9, 93, 94–5, *95*, 160; use of
  term, 3n1. *See also* Indigenous
  adolescents; Indigenous children,
  with respiratory challenges;
  Indigenous parents and
  caregivers
Indigenous Youth Mentorship
  Program, 98–9, 99–100
interdisciplinary collaboration, 12,
  164–5, 166
International Association for Public
  Participation, 96
International Organization for
  Migration (IOM), 66
International Society for Social
  Paediatrics and Child Health, 60
intersectionality, 26

intimate partner (domestic) violence, 31, 152, 153
Inuit, 32, 99. *See also* Indigenous peoples
isolation. *See* social isolation

John F. Kennedy University, 163

King, Alexandra, 99
knowledge: Indigenous parents and, 140; influence on other programs and services, 163; low-income parents and, 127, 130; obsessive-compulsive disorder and, 58; professional and experiential, 160–1; respiratory challenges and, 22, 85; for service providers about life challenges, 161–2
knowledge translation: about, 11, 12, 122, 150; at end-of-study, 154–6; engaging knowledge users, 150–2; impacts and implications, 156–8; in intervention research processes, 152–4

Lancet, The, 5
learning, in peer support groups, 110–11
loneliness. *See* social isolation
Loneliness and Social Dissatisfaction Questionnaire for Young Children, 89
Longitudinal Study of Child Development in Quebec, 33
low income, 83, 123–4
low-income adolescents, with respiratory challenges: about, 11, 81, 83–4; insights and implications, 91; methodology of studies, 84–5, 87–8; support interventions, impacts of, 88–90; support needs and preferences, 85–7

low-income parents and caregivers: about, 121, 123–4, 134; childcare and transportation challenges, 126; communication with, 131; community outreach and, 132; coping strategies and, 129–30; discriminatory health care interactions, 127; environment and education barriers, 127; financial stress, 125–6, 159; isolation and, 129; knowledge and, 130, 153; medication challenges, 125–6; methodological approach, 124–5; proactive support for, 132–4; service providers and, 130–4; support for accessing resources, 131–2; support gaps and stressors, 125–8; support intervention impacts, 129–30; support intervention program, 128–9, 133–4, 162; support preferences, 127–8

major depressive disorder, 44, 50, 51. *See also* depression
Marshall, Albert, 95
McGavock, Jon, 98
medication: education about, 127, 130; financial coverage, 23, 124, 125–6, 141; knowledge gaps, 85, 140; for obsessive-compulsive disorder, 56; respiratory challenges and, 85, 86, 89
mental health, adolescents and children: about, 11, 15–16, 29–30, 64–5, 159–60; food insecurity and, 33; future research priorities, 64; geography and, 32–3; housing and homelessness, 32; immigrants and, 15, 33–5, 67–9; improving access to service, 62–3; Indigenous peoples and, 35–6,

mental health ... (*cont'd*)
   61, 92; prevalence, 29; social and
   environmental risk factors, 36–7;
   socio-economic inequalities and,
   30–1; targeting social inequalities
   and determinants for improving,
   59–61; treatment and social risks,
   62. *See also* African immigrant
   children, and mental health;
   obsessive-compulsive disorder
Mental Health Commission of
   Canada (MHCC), 60, 63, 68
mental health literacy, 58
Métis. *See* Indigenous peoples
migrants, 3n2, 7, 66. *See also*
   immigrants; refugees
Mi'kmaq peoples, 138, 143
Mi'kmaw Ethics Watch, 138
mindfulness-based intervention, 52, 55
mood disorders, 34, 59, 67
Mothers Offering Mentorship and
   Support (MOMS) Link, 151–2,
   156, 158
multiculturalism, 107
Multidimensional Scale of Perceived
   Social Support, 90

National Allergy Strategy:
   AllergyMATE, 163
National Anxiety Disorders Screening
   Day, 58
National Population Health Survey, 68
natural disaster, 31
New Canadian Children and Youth
   Study, 34
newcomers, 3n2, 159, 160. *See also*
   immigrants; migrants; refugees
nurses, 144–5

obesity, 98
obsessive-compulsive disorder
   (OCD): about, 29–30, 37–8, 64–5;
academic skills and, 51–2; adverse
   childhood experiences and, 43, *48*;
   biology and pathophysiology of,
   42; cognitive behavioural therapy
   and, 54, 56, 57; co-morbidities,
   50; culture and, 39–40, *48*;
   definition, 37; determinants of
   health affected by, 43, *44*; disease
   trajectory, 43–5; epidemiology of,
   38–9; ethnicity and, 39–40, *48*,
   58–9; family accommodation and,
   49, 53–4; family communication
   and, *49*; family's role in treatment,
   54–5; functional implications,
   50–1; gender and, *47*; geography
   and rural residence, 39, *47*, *48*, 53;
   heritability of, 42; impact on family,
   53; improving access to services,
   63; income and, *47*, 50; Indigenous
   peoples and, 41–2; interventions
   and inequalities in, 55–9; lack of
   knowledge about, 58; medications
   for, 56; parental education and,
   47; prevalence, 39; quality of life
   and, 51; residential treatment,
   56–7; sleep and, 46; social and
   familial risk factors, 42–3; social
   determinants of health affecting,
   43, *45*, *47–9*; socio-economic factors
   and, 39, 40–1, *47*; stressful life event
   and, *49*, 56; suicide and, 46, 49;
   symptoms, 45–6; treatment barriers,
   57–9; treatment overview, 56–7
Obsessive Compulsive Disorder
   Collaborative Genetics Association
   Study, 50
OCD Family Functioning Scale, 53
oneHealth, 142, 144
online support programs, 63,
   162, 165. *See also* computer
   skills; Indigenous children, with
   respiratory challenges; Indigenous

parents and caregivers; low-income adolescents, with respiratory challenges; low-income parents and caregivers; social media; Syrian refugee adolescents
Ontario Child Health Study, 31
oppositional defiant disorder, 30, 44, 50

parents, 121–2. *See also* families; Indigenous parents and caregivers; knowledge translation; low-income parents and caregivers; postpartum depression; refugee new parents
participatory action research (PAR), 9, 10, 95
participatory research, community-based, 9, 10, 137, 151
Pediatric Quality of Life Enjoyment and Satisfaction Questionnaire, 51
peer-support interventions, 9, 148, 151–2, 162–3. *See also* Indigenous children, with respiratory challenges; Indigenous parents and caregivers; low-income adolescents, with respiratory challenges; low-income parents and caregivers; Syrian refugee adolescents
Personal Resource Questionnaire, 143
pharmaceuticals. *See* medication
Philadelphia Neurodevelopmental Cohort, 41
physical abuse, 31
physical illness/injury, 31
postpartum depression, 151–2, 155, 156, 157, 158
post-traumatic stress disorder, 34, 70
poverty. *See* income and poverty; low-income adolescents, with respiratory challenges; low-income parents and caregivers
prescription drugs. *See* medication

Proactive Coping Inventory, 143
psychology, community, 36
psychosis, 32
public participation, 9, 12, 164–5. *See also* Ethical Space; participatory action research; participatory research, community-based; strengths-based approaches; Two-eyed Seeing
purposive sampling, 84, 124

quality of life, and obsessive-compulsive disorder (OCD), 51
queer youth, 36

race. *See* ethnicity
racism: academic skills and, 51; African immigrants and, 70–2, 75–6; Indigenous children with respiratory challenges and, 19, 22–3, 26, 27, 49
refugee new parents, 70, 151, 153, 156, 161
refugees: in Canada, 101; challenges facing, 101–2, 159; children as, 66; definition, 3n2; increase in, 7; low income and, 123; marginalization of, 7; mental health and, 34; strengths-based approach and, 164; Syrian refugees in Canada, 103. *See also* African immigrant children, and mental health; refugee new parents; Syrian refugee adolescents
relationship building, 108–9, 112–13, 160
research methodologies: about, 9–11; community-based participatory research, 9, 10, 137, 151; Ethical Space, 93–4, *94*; participatory action research, 9, 10, 95; purposive sampling, 84, 124; snowball sampling, 20;

research methodologies (*cont'd*)
strengths-based approaches, 9, 10,
95–7, *97*, 164; Two-eyed Seeing
(*Etuaptmumk*), 9, 93, 94–5, *95*, 160
residential treatment, for obsessive-
compulsive disorder (OCD), 56–7
resilience, 8, 96–7, 116–17, 164
respiratory system diseases, 18. *See
also* Indigenous children, with
respiratory challenges; Indigenous
parents and caregivers; low-income
adolescents, with respiratory
challenges; low-income parents
and caregivers
rural residence. *See* geography and
rural residence

school system, 22–3, 71, 73–4, 107
serotonin reuptake inhibitor
medications, 56
service providers: communication
and, 131; community outreach
and, 132; discrimination and,
127; engagement with Indigenous
peoples, 144–7, 148–9; knowledge
considerations, 160–2; partnerships
with other organizations, 163;
proactive support and, 132–4;
support from accessing
resources, 131
sexual abuse, 31
sexually transmitted diseases, 92, 99
sexual-related minority youth, 36
sharing experiences, 109–10
single-parent families, 34, 123
sleep, 46
smoking, 23, 85, 140
snowball sampling, 20
social comparison theory, 9, 113
social determinants of health:
about, 5, 163–5; future directions,
166–7; Indigenous, 36, 92; mental

health in children and, 30–3,
36–7; newcomers and, 160; World
Health Organization on, 62. *See
also* culture; ethnicity; geography
and rural residence; income and
poverty; social support
social exchange theory, 9, 113
social isolation (social exclusion):
about, 3, 8, 160; adolescent
newcomers, 113, 115; African
immigrant children, 73–4;
Indigenous parents, 140, 143; low-
income parents, 129; respiratory
challenges and, 21–2, 85–6, 87, 89,
91; support interventions for, 162–3
social learning, 9, 113
social media, 112, 155–6
social support, 3, 5, 8–9, 162–3. *See also*
peer-support interventions
socio-economic factors: future
research directions, 165–6; mental
health in children and, 30–1;
obsessive-compulsive disorder and,
39, 40–1, *47*; respiratory challenges
and, 86, 124. *See also* income and
poverty
South Asian Canadians, 61
speech and language disorders, 50
stigma: African immigrants and
mental health, 74; Indigenous
parents, 140; mental health and,
40, 42, 60–1; reduction of, 147,
162; respiratory challenges and,
21, 91
Strategy for Patient-Oriented
Research, 96
street-entrenched youth. *See*
homelessness
strengths-based approaches, 9, 10,
95–7, *97*, 164
stressful life events, and obsessive-
compulsive disorder (OCD), *49*, 56

Sudanese refugees. *See* refugee new parents
suicide, 29, 46, 49
support, seeking, 111
Sykes Telecare, 158
Syrian refugee adolescents: about, 8, 11–12, 82, 102–3; implications for other refugee adolescent programs, 115–17; initial experiences in Canada, 106–8; learning and, 110–11; relationship building and, 108–9, 112–13, 160; seeking support and, 111; sharing experiences and, 109–10; support intervention program, content, 111–13; support intervention program, development, 103–5; support intervention program, evaluation methods, 105–6; support intervention program, impacts, 113–14, 115; support intervention program, theoretical basis, 113; support intervention program, youths' experiences, 108–11

Tafoya, Terry, 95
technology skills, 104, 115–16, 128. *See also* online support programs; social media
Telehealth, 142, 144
telephone cognitive behavioural therapy, 63
tics, 37, 50
traditional medicines, 141
transportation, 22, 126, 140–1, 142

trauma: colonialism and, 35, 98; pre-emigration, 69–70, 75; refugees and, 101–2; trauma-based, resilience-informed model of Indigenous health, *97*
Two-eyed Seeing (*Etuaptmumk*), 9, 94–5, *95*, 160
Two-Row Wampum Belt Treaty (1613), 94

UCLA Loneliness Scale, 129, 143
UK Millennium Cohort Study, 31
underdiagnosis, 141
United Nations Declaration on the Rights of Indigenous Peoples, 96

wage discrimination, 71
wellness, 96–7
Williams, D.R., 27
World Health Organization (WHO): Commission on Social Determinants of Health, 8; *Global Plan of Action on Social Determinants of Health*, 62; on Indigenous children and health inequalities, 17; on obsessive-compulsive disorder, 29

youth, 81–2. *See also* Indigenous adolescents; low-income adolescents, with respiratory challenges; mental health, adolescents and children; Syrian refugee adolescents

Zimbabwean refugees. *See* refugee new parents